Practical Research Methods for Physiother

Fiona Collen
Rivermead, Oxford
August 1989

For my parents

Practical Research Methods for Physiotherapists

Carolyn M. Hicks BA MA PhD CertEd ABPsS

Lecturer in Psychology, Department of Extramural Studies, University of Birmingham, Birmingham, UK

CHURCHILL LIVINGSTONE

EDINBURGH LONDON MELBOURNE AND NEW YORK 1988

CHURCHILL LIVINGSTONE
Medical Division of Longman Group UK Limited

Distributed in the United States of America by
Churchill Livingstone Inc., 1560 Broadway, New
York, N.Y. 10036, and by associated companies,
branches and representatives throughout the world.

First published 1988

ISBN 0-443-03757-4

British Library Cataloguing in Publication, Data
Hicks, Carolyn
    Practical research methods for
    physiotherapists.
    1. Physical therapy—Research—
    Methodology
    I. Title
    001.4'024615   RM708

Library of Congress Cataloging in Publication Data
Hicks, Carolyn.
    Practical research methods for physiotherapists.
    Bibliography: p.
    Includes index.
    1. Physical therapy—Research—Statistical
    methods.
I. Title.
RM708.H53   198   615.8'2'072   87–18383

Produced by Longman Singapore Publishers Pte Ltd
Printed in Singapore

Preface

The purpose of this book, quite simply, is to provide any physiotherapist who is thinking of doing some research, with the necessary tools to complete the task. Research methods and statistics are not the most inherently entertaining of topics; to put it bluntly, the majority of students find the subject as dull as ditchwater. However, if the subject can be seen as a means to a much more interesting end, then most people are prepared to tolerate the tedium of working through the essential issues, in the knowledge that the practical application of the theory can be very exciting, as well as potentially useful to their profession.

While there are numerous books on research methods and statistical analysis currently available, this book differs in a number of respects. Firstly, it is not written by a statistician, but by someone who still occasionally goes blank at the sight of a page of new formulae. This, I hope, means that I may be more aware of some of the fundamental difficulties that many people experience when confronted with numbers.

Undoubtedly, many students have a mental block when it comes to maths of any sort. Whatever the origin of this, it is important to recognise that this block is much more likely to be emotional rather than intellectual in nature. In an attempt to overcome any potential problems relating to this, I have tried to make the book as readable and non-jargon oriented as possible.

Secondly, very little statistical theory has been included here. The majority of books on research methods and statistics provide particularly detailed theoretical accounts of how individual statistical formulae have been derived. Such a level of explanation tends to confuse and discourage many aspiring researchers. In consequence, the student often fails to grasp even the basic principles. While acknowledging the importance of such a full understanding, this text takes the view that a practical, readily available guide to designing research programmes in terms of sound scientific principles, as well as to choosing the appropriate form of analysis for the results is more effective.

It should be pointed out, however, that the statistical analyses covered in this book are by no means exhaustive. Many more complex statistical techniques are available should the research warrant them, and these can be found in more advanced texts. A cautionary note, though. Different terminology is used in different statistics' texts, and you may need to cross check the indexes of books for compatible terms.

And finally, the focus of the book is research in *physiotherapy*. I have taught numerous courses on statistics and research methods for various members of the paramedical professions and it seems to me that the most successful way of presenting a new concept is by making it directly relevant to the experience of the learners. If the examples and situations quoted are familiar to the audience, then the chances of a new idea being understood are optimised. That having been said, I'm not a physiotherapist either, and so you may find some of the examples fairly ludicrous. If you don't, then it is due entirely to Doreen Caney, Principal of the Queen Elizabeth School of Physiotherapy in Birmingham to whom I am indebted. She has furnished me with numerous ideas, guidance, information and help; without her, the book would not have been started in the first place, and nor would it have been completed. If inaccurate statements about physiotherapy remain in the text, it is because I misused her advice. Sincerest thanks are due to her. Secondly, I wish to thank my excellent secretary, Janet Francis, who ploughed her way through my appalling maze of a manuscript with consummate skill and good humour. Thanks are also due to Christine O'Donoghue and Christine Marshall who were prime movers and facilitators in getting this project off the ground. And lastly, I owe a great deal to my husband, Dr Peter Spurgeon, for his invaluable comments on the theoretical content of the book and the lucidity of its presentation.

Birmingham 1988   Carolyn M. Hicks

Acknowledgements

I am indebted to the following sources for granting permission to reproduce the statistical tables in Appendix 2 of this book:

Tables A2.1, A2.5 and A2.6 from Lindley D V, Miller J C P 1973 Cambridge Elementary Statistical Tables, 10th edn. Cambridge University Press, Cambridge

Table A2.2 from Wilcoxon F, Wilcox R A 1949 Some Rapid Approximate Statistical Procedures. American Cyanamid Company
Reproduced with the permission of the American Cyanamid Company.

Table A2.3 from Friedman M 1937 The use of ranks to avoid the assumptions of normality implicit in the analysis of variance. Journal of the American Statistical Association 32

Table A2.4 from Page E E 1963 in the Journal of the American Statistical Association 58

Table A2.7 from Runyon R P, Haber A 1976 Fundamentals of Behavioural Statistics 3rd edn. Addison Wesley, Reading Mass

Table A2.8 from Kruskal W H, Wallis W A 1952 The use of ranks in one-criterion variance analysis. Journal of the American Statistical Association 47

Table A2.9 from Jonckheere A R 1954 A distribution-free k-sample test against ordered alternatives. Biometrika 14 (Biometrika Trustees)

Table A2.10 from Olds E G 1949 The 5% significance levels for sums of squares of rank differences and a correction. Annals of Mathematical Statistics 20 (The Institute of Mathematical Statistics)

Table A2.11 from Table VII (p. 63) of Fisher R A, Yates F 1974 Statistical Tables for Biological, Agricultural and Medical Research. Longman Group Ltd, London (previously published by Oliver and Boyd Ltd, Edinburgh). I am grateful to the Literary Executor of the late Sir Ronald Fisher, F.R.S., to Dr Frank Yates and to Longman Group Ltd,

London for permission to reprint Table VII from their book Statistical Tables for Biological, Agricultural and Medical Research, 6th edn. 1974

Table A2.12 adapted from Friedman M 1940 A comparison of alternative tests of significance for the problem of m rankings. Annals of Mathematical Statistics

Contents

1

Introduction

THE NEED FOR RESEARCH IN PHYSIOTHERAPY

Why carry out research in physiotherapy? Surely the profession is sufficiently well-established to make such activities irrelevant — after all, many of the therapeutic techniques currently in practice have been developed over the years and consequently are tried and tested. Is there *really* any need to start introducing experiments and statistical analysis?

I have heard these arguments on a number of occasions and have some sympathy with this point of view. However, as I have written this book on experimental design and statistics for physiotherapy, it must be apparent that my opinion does not accord with this stance. While this is no place to enter the debate, I would like to outline briefly why I feel that research is fundamental to the profession.

My first argument is a general one. There is an increasing trend towards physiotherapy becoming a graduate profession and those degree courses currently in operation all have a heavy science component. Nor is this inappropriate, since physiotherapy is clearly scientific in content. However, all sciences have at their root, a reliance on experimentation, data collection and statistical analysis. If physiotherapy is to submit to the scientific rigour inherent in a degree course, it must incorporate research methodology and statistics. Such a component lends credibility, not only academically, but professionally. Furthermore, an understanding of research methods and statistics allows the physiotherapist to evaluate other professionals' research activities and reports.

The second point in favour of research in physiotherapy relates to much more specific problem-driven issues. There are many physiotherapists who, at the risk of disagreement from their colleagues, would admit that many of the therapeutic procedures they use are selected on the basis of intuition, personal preference and familiarity, rather than on the basis of empirically established information. To illustrate this point, consider the following problem issues:

1. You are about to treat a recent injury where pain is the predominant symptom. Do you select ice or ultrasound? Why? When I asked the same

question of a group of highly trained physiotherapists, their opinion was divided. While this could suggest that both methods are equally effective, in this instance I do not think this was the case. Every member of the group put forward an argument for one or other treatment *based on his/her own experience* and not on any research evidence. In other words, their views were divided because treatment selection was a matter of opinion and not of hard factual evidence deriving from experimentation. Research in areas like this might compare the relative outcome of different types of treatment, thus removing the subjective element and making the decision process clearer, less ambiguous and hopefully more effective.

2. The uniform/no uniform issue continues to be contentious in some quarters. There are sound arguments on both sides, the pro-uniform lobby claiming that the uniform inspires greater confidence and trust in the patient, while the anti-uniform contingent argues that it decreases rapport. So how can the issue be resolved? The answer lies in the use of experimental method and statistical analysis — if the effects of wearing uniform vs wearing 'civvies' are measured and analysed using scientific techniques, the debate can be settled.

3. You are presented with a new piece of apparatus for treating frozen shoulders. Do you try it on the first patient who comes along and then, depending on whether the outcome *appears* to show some effects, order half a dozen more? Or do you set up a controlled experiment whereby you systematically compare the effectiveness of the new apparatus with the effectiveness of the standard treatment procedure? If you opted for the latter you will need a sound knowledge of scientific methodology and data analysis.

I hope that you can see from these examples of problem-driven issues that experimentation and statistical analysis are essential if physiotherapeutic procedures are to be systematised and optimised. In the current era of increasing pressure on resources, hit and miss policies of treatment based on opinion and preference rather than hard evidence are too wasteful of time and money to be justified. Therefore it is crucial for physiotherapists to evaluate their procedures systematically to make the profession even more efficient, cost-effective and successful. To do this, a knowledge of experimental design, research methods and statistical analysis is essential.

A final caveat — I am not a physiotherapist — a point which will doubtless become clear to you as you read this book. As a result I tend to make physiotherapy up as I go along, so if there are examples which strike you as ludicrous, naïve or just impossible, please forgive me.

USING STATISTICS

Statistics are a crucial part of research. Whenever someone carries out an experiment it is essential that the results are analysed and presented in a way that can be understood by other interested parties. Statistics are the means by which this is achieved. For example, if an experiment had been carried out to compare ultrasound with accessory movements in treating arthritic toe joints, it is insufficient just to present a table of figure showing range of movement for each patient following treatment and expecting the reader to make sense of it. The data has to be analysed and interpreted using statistical methods, so that an objective conclusion can be reached in terms of which of the two treatments is better.

However, many people are put off research *because* of the statistical procedures that are required. They see a page of formulae and figures, panic and slam the book shut. This suggests the first and most important rule of statistics — **do not panic**! Inability to understand statistics is rarely an intellectual problem, but an *emotional* one, and anyone who feels diffident in the face of figures should remember this. As long as you approach the statistical analysis systematically and in a step-by-step manner, there should be few problems.

Another point should be raised here. Do not imagine that the object of statistical analysis is to test your long multiplication and division — it isn't. Statistics are no more than a tool for analysing data. So, always use a calculator—it is quicker and usually more reliable than even the quickest mind.

And lastly, remember that you don't need to memorise formulae — as long as you know where to look them up and how to use them there is no need to commit them to memory. Further, at the risk of being hammered by the purists, I would also add that there is no need to understand *how* the formula was derived from statistical theory. While many statisticians would vehemently disagree with that rather bald statement, I would liken statistical analysis to any other tool or piece of apparatus — you don't need to understand the workings of a car or television in order to use it. If that were the case, only garage mechanics would be allowed to drive cars. Many would argue, of course, that if you *do* understand the mechanism, then you are able to put it right if the apparatus goes wrong. However, if you know *when, why* and *how* to use a statistical method, and if you follow the procedure step-by-step, then the statistical tool will not break down. It is the when, why and how of statistics that this book aims to explain.

STRUCTURE OF THE BOOK

The book has been divided into sections which are devoted to designing experiments and to statistical procedures. I would recommend that anyone who feels unsure of themselves mathematically should read Appendix 1 at the end of the book. The rest of you may wish just to refresh your memories on some basic rules of mathematics. These are presented briefly in the next section. Once you have read as far as Chapter 6 you *should* have a sound idea of how to design experiments and which analysis to use on any data resulting from them. After that point, the chapters are devoted to outlining the procedures involved in particular statistical tests. You should read the relevant chapter as and when required. For this reason, these chapters are independent of each other and so may contain common material. I make no apologies for this repetition, since I find nothing more irritating than to open a statistics book at the relevant chapter only to discover that certain essential elements have been covered earlier, necessitating the reading of additional chapters in which I have little immediate interest. For this reason, the chapters on statistical tests are virtually self-contained.

Throughout the book, too, there are exercises to test your understanding of a particular principle. If you decide to do these, you will find the answers at the back of the book. Also, within each chapter, at appropriate intervals, there are 'Key Concept' boxes, which summarise the most important points. These can be used to refresh your memory without having to plough through pages of typescript to find what you want.

Finally, there aren't a lot of laughs in statistics. Many students find the topic dry, so I've tried to make the style as chatty as possible. Nonetheless, jokes are hard to come by, but do persevere — statistics are an essential part of research life.

So, I hope you will find that this book equips you with the basic elements you need for your research. Happy experimenting!

P.S. All the experiments and data in the book are entirely fictitious!

P.P.S. Please note that all the calculations in the examples and activities have been worked to three decimal places throughout.

SOME BASIC MATHS

Most of us have forgotten many of the basic mathematical concepts we learnt for 'O'-level, simply because we don't use them very often. Even though you are advised to use a calculator to compute the statistical tests in this book, it is still essential that you are familiar with the basic mathematical principles, for two main reasons. Firstly, even though a calculator will do all the most complex multiplying, dividing and square-rooting for you, you will need to know the *order* in which these processes are carried out, because, as you will no doubt remember, some types of computation must be done before others. This will be clarified later. Secondly, even though you will be using a calculator, it is still quite possible to come up with some odd results, either because some information has been entered wrongly, or simply because on occasions, calculators have been known to go haywire. So you need to be able to 'eyeball' the results of your calculations to see if they *look* right. If you have any doubts or reservations about any of this, read on.

This section is just a brief reminder of some of the basic principles you will need. These principles are discussed in greater detail in Appendix 1, so if you are unsure of any of them, turn to page 247.

Some basic rules

1. If the formula contains brackets, you must carry out all the calculations inside them first.
2. If the formula contains brackets within brackets, you must do the calculations in the innermost brackets first.
3. If the formula contains no brackets, do the multiplications and divisions first.
4. If the formula contains only additions and substractions, work from left to right.
5. Adding two negative numbers results in a negative answer.
6. Adding a plus number to a minus number is the same as taking the minus number from the plus number.
7. Multiplying two positive numbers gives a positive answer.
8. Multiplying a positive number and a negative number together gives a negative answer.
9. Multiplying two negative numbers gives a positive answer.
10. Dividing a positive number by a negative number (or vice versa) gives a negative answer.
11. Dividing two negative numbers gives a positive answer.
12. The square of a number is that number multiplied by itself. It is expressed as ^{2}.
13. The square root of a given number is a number which when multiplied by itself gives the number you already have. It is expressed as $\sqrt{\ }$.
14. To round up decimal points, start at the extreme right hand number. If it is 5 or more, increase the number to its left by 1. If it is less than 5, the number to its left remains the same.

You might like to do the following exercises just to satisfy yourself that you're happy with these rules.

Activity I (Answers on page 271)

Calculate the following:

1. $14 + 8 + 27 - 3$
2. $14 + 8 - (27 - 3)$
3. $17 + (30 - 4)$
4. $11 (19 + 4)$
5. $19 \times 3 + 8$
6. $12 + (14 \times 3) - 5$
7. $6 [(4 + 8) - 3]$
8. $15 - 4 \times 4 + 12$
9. $(49 - 1) + 7 \times 8$
10. $36 - (12 - 6) + 17$
11. $- 18 + 22 - 10$
12. $- 24 + 16$
13. $- 12 \times +4$
14. $+ 18 - 26$
15. $- 14 \times -3$
16. $- 51 + 3$

17. $51 - (+ 3 \times + 2)$
18. $+ 17 - 4 - 26$
19. $- 19 + 11 + 15$
20. $- 5 (4 \times 12)$

SYMBOLS IN STATISTICS

You will find the following symbols appearing in formulae throughout the book. Although they will be explained when they appear, this page can serve as a quick reference point.

Σ = sum or total of all the calculations to the right of the symbol
  e.g. $\Sigma 3^2 + 6^2 + 4^2 = 61$

x = an individual score

$\bar{x}$ = the average score

$\sqrt{}$ = the square root of a figure or calculations,
  e.g. $\sqrt{89} = 9.434$
  $\sqrt{17 + 15 + 86} = 10.863$
  $\sqrt{51 \times 3} + 4 = 12.37 + 4$
  $\phantom{\sqrt{51 \times 3} + 4} = 16.369$

N = the total number of scores in an experiment

^{2} = the number times itself,
  e.g. $8^2 = 8 \times 8$
  $ = 64$

$<$ = less than,
  e.g. $5 < 7$ (5 is less than 7)

$>$ = more than,
  e.g. $10 > 2$ (10 is more than 2)

C = the number of conditions in the experiment

n = the number of scores in a sub-group or condition.

2

Approaches to statistics

Whenever you engage in research, you will end up *measuring* something — muscle tone, recovery rate, vital capacity, numbers of patients, etc. These measurements are called *data*. In order for the research to have some value, the meaning of this data has to be presented in ways that other research workers can understand. For example, there is no point in carrying out a well-designed experiment to compare the effectiveness of two bladder control techniques in multiple sclerosis sufferers, if the data on this is just left a jumbled mass of figures. In other words, the researcher has to *make sense* of the results.

There are various ways of making sense of the results, but for the physiotherapist two methods are of major importance. The first approach is called **descriptive statistics**, whereby the researcher collects a set of data, usually from a form of *survey* and then describes it in terms of its most important features, e.g. average scores, range of scores etc.; the second approach is called **inferential statistics** in which the data, which has usually been collected from an *experiment*, is subject to statistical analysis using tests which allow the researcher to make inferences beyond the actual data in front of him/her. The differences between these approaches will be discussed briefly now, and then later in more detail.

DESCRIPTIVE STATISTICS

As has already been mentioned, descriptive statistics are usually used in conjunction with survey methods. Surveys involve collecting a large quantity of data on a particular topic and analysing it using techniques of descriptive statistics to emphasise some of its more interesting features.

Let's take an example. Supposing you are interested in the general topic of community physiotherapy. You could easily gather a vast quantity of data on this topic, e.g.

1. the number of community physiotherapists currently employed in a particular district and their specialities
2. the number of calls made on average per week within the district over the last year

3. the types of patients seen (their ages, ethnic origin, social class, sex, etc.) over the last year
4. the average amount of time spent treating a particular category of patient
5. any changes in the execution of community physiotherapy over the previous 10-year period could be noted, e.g. any increase in provision to a particular patient group.

From all this survey data, you could gain the following sorts of information:

— what is going on in a particular area (type and extent of community physiotherapy service provision)
— identification of areas of existing or potential problems (e.g. lesser provision in some geographical areas or for some categories of patient)
— measurement of the extent of these problems
— the generation of possible explanations for them.

In addition to all this, the survey could identify past trends and so could be used to predict future patterns (e.g. with the population growth in the over-75 age group, and the increasing trend towards community-based care, the need for greater provision of community physiotherapists with a special interest in geriatric problems would be highlighted).

The outcome of such surveys can radically influence major, as well as minor, policy decisions. And if such policy changes are implemented, survey techniques may be used to evaluate the impact these changes have. (For further information on survey methods see Gardner (1978).) It might be useful at this point to look at some of the ways in which descriptive statistics might be useful to the physiotherapist, by means of a more specific illustration.

Suppose that you are the principal of a school of physiotherapy. Obviously, in this role you will be concerned about the standards of student performance, both clinical and theoretical, in your school. In particular, you may want to find out (a) whether these standards are dropping or rising from year to year and (b) how they compare with other schools throughout the country. To do this you need to employ some common mathematical techniques in order to highlight certain features of the data, in other words, descriptive statistics. Let's take the first example. To find out whether the standards are changing from year to year, you could take the *average* mark in both final theory and clinical exams over, say, the last 10 years. From this you can draw a graph to get the general picture of the standards of performance. You might end up with something like this:

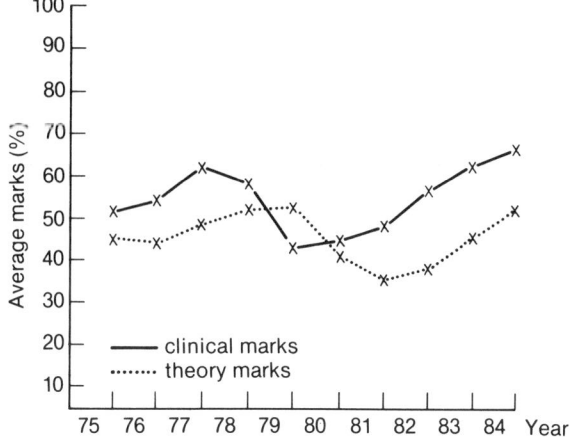

Fig. 1 Average clinical and theory marks over the past 10 years in a school of physiotherapy.

From such a graph of *average* marks, you can get the general picture of the trend of performance and also the comparative performance on clinical and theory exams.

To solve your second problem of how your school compares with others, you can collect the average marks from all the other schools for 1984, and compare yours with these. You might obtain the following data:

School	Average theory mark	Average clinical mark
A	63%	58%
B	45%	55%
C	48%	59%
D	57%	45%
E	70%	50%
F	52%	60%
G	54%	61%
H	67%	66%

Your own averages (66% for theory, 52% for clinical — see Fig. 1) can be compared with the other schools to find out how well your school does. It can be seen, then, from this information that your school comes 3rd in the theory exams, but only 7th in the clinical exams. From the above information, too, you can see that although school E has the best marks on theory, they have the biggest discrepancy between theory and practice, while school H appears to be the most consistent. In other words, you can glean a considerable amount of information from such data.

It should be pointed out that there are many ways of describing your data besides the methods illustrated above. However the three most commonly used forms of descriptive statistics are *graphs, measures of central tendency*, which present data in terms of the most typical scores and results, and *measures of dispersion*, which present data in terms of the variation in the scores. Each of these will be discussed in the section entitled 'Techniques of descriptive statistics.'

Descriptive statistics, then, are used when the researcher has collected a large quantity of data, usually from a survey of some sort, and wishes to extract certain sorts of information from it in order to provide a description of the data. It is important to recognise that descriptive statistics allow you to make statements about features of your data that are of interest but they do not allow you to *infer* anything beyond the results you have in front of you. In other words, if you were measuring the muscle tone of a group of 20 muscular dystrophy patients, you could use descriptive statistics to make statements about the muscle tone data of *that particular group* of patients in terms of average tone, range of tone, speed of contractions etc. What you could *not* do would be to infer anything about the muscle tone of muscular dystrophy patients *as a whole* simply on the basis of the data from your particular group. To be able to do that you have to use techniques called *inferential statistics*.

INFERENTIAL STATISTICS

Prior to every election, we are bombarded with the results of opinion polls which tell us how well one political party is likely to do compared with the others. In order to obtain this sort of information, a *sample* of the general public is questioned, since it would be impossible to ask the opinions of every member of the electorate. From the responses given by this sample, the attitudes of the rest of the voters are estimated, or *inferred*. However, we all know that these opinion polls may be quite incorrect. For example, if the opinion pollsters *only* went to a polo match in Surrey and asked the views of the spectators, they would be likely to get a very different picture of the prevailing political opinion than if they *only* went to a rugby match in South Wales. In other words, if the opinion poll is to have any value in predicting the outcome of an election, the sample of potential voters selected for the poll must be representative of the population as a whole and not representative of just one section of it.

The usual method of selecting a sample which is representative of the population from which it is drawn is a technique called *random sampling*. For a sample to be random, it must have been selected in such a way that every member of the relevant population had an equal chance of being chosen. For example, if 6 playing cards are to be randomly selected from a pack, the pack is first shuffled and any 6 cards are chosen. Assuming the dealer did not hide any or keep his thumb on some, then these 6 cards will be a random sample because every one of the 52 cards had an equal chance of selection. Now, there are two important points here. Firstly, if these cards are not replaced and a second random sample is drawn from the same population, it will not be the same; so, if another set of 6 cards is selected from the pack, they will be different from the first set because there is only one Ace of Clubs, Seven of Hearts etc. in a pack. Similarly, any two groups of hysterectomy patients, if randomly drawn from a population of hysterectomy patients, will not be identical in their characteristics (age, height, fitness etc.) Secondly, the larger the random sample drawn, the more likely it is that it will be fairly representative of the population from which it comes. So, a random sample of 3 hysterectomy patients out of a total population of 60 will stand less chance of being representative than a random sample of 35. Information about the ways in which the researcher can select a random sample *in practice* are given in Chapter 4. Returning to the opinion poll, even if the sample *is* representative of the whole population, there will still be an element of error in the predictions about the election (because some voters subsequently change their views, fail to vote or misunderstand the questions etc.).

Nonetheless, if the voters selected for the poll have been chosen randomly, according to certain statistical principles, then this degree of error can be calculated using a branch of statistics known as *inferential statistics*. Essentially what this approach enables the researcher to do is to select a small sample of people for study, and from the results of that study to make inferences about the population from which that sample was drawn. Usually, the way in which this is done is by formulating an hypothesis, setting up an experiment to test the hypothesis and using inferential statistics to analyse the results of your experiment to see if your hypothesis has been supported. In other words, inferential statistics are used in testing hypotheses. It should be pointed out at this stage, that there are two main types of research design which are used to test hypotheses: *experimental designs* and *correlational designs*. They will be described in detail in the next chapter.

One classic way in which the physiotherapist might use this approach is in the comparison of different treatment techniques with patients. Let's suppose you were interested in trying to establish bladder control among middle-aged women suffering stress incontinence. You have two techniques, A and B, and you want to find out which is more effective. For a host of practical reasons, you cannot test every middle-aged women with stress incontinence, and so you select a *random* sample of, say, 20 women and assign them to Treatment A and a further random sample of 20 women and assign them to Treatment B. Both groups are treated in exactly the same way except for the nature of their treatment, and at the end of a given period, you compare the groups in terms of bladder control. Suppose you find that the incidence of stress incontinence is less (i.e. improved) for Treatment A group than for Treatment B. Now you would expect that there would be *some* differences between the groups anyway, simply because of chance factors, like the mood swings of the patients, personality factors, current state of health, fatigue etc. but the question is whether the difference between the two groups in terms of the incidence of stress incontinence can be accounted for by these chance factors, or whether the difference is due to the relative effectiveness of the treatments. If the experiment has been carried out properly and in accordance with certain prerequisite conditions (see Chs. 3, 4, and 5 for details on this), then statistical tests can be used to analyse the data and to conclude whether the difference between the groups is, in fact, attributable to the type of treatment or not. If it is found to be due to the treatment procedure, then you would conclude that Treatment A is more effective with this group. If you have selected your sample of patients randomly from middle-aged women with stress incontinence *as a whole*, then you could reasonably *infer* that Treatment A is likely to be more effective than Treatment B with other sufferers, and hence you would recommend it to other physiotherapists. In other words, you have selected a small sample for study and from the results of this study, you can make inferences about the whole population from which the sample was drawn. This is the basis of inferential statistics.

Key concepts

Data from research must be presented in a way that can be understood by the reader. There are two main ways of doing this:

- Descriptive statistics, which summarise the main features of the results from a survey by describing the average scores etc.
- Inferential statistics which are used to test hypotheses and which involve selecting a small sample of people for study and from the results of this, allowing the researcher to make inferences about the population from which the sample was drawn.

In other words, descriptive statistics allow the researcher to make statements *only* about the results obtained, but do not permit any assumptions to be made beyond the data collected, whereas inferential statistics allow the researcher to make assumptions *beyond* the set of data in front of her/him.

TECHNIQUES OF DESCRIPTIVE STATISTICS

Graphs

Sometimes it is easier to make sense of a set of data if it is presented as a graph rather than as a table of results. While a graph tells you no more than a table of figures, it often shows trends and other features of the data more clearly. Since we have all drawn graphs in school and elsewhere, the principles pertaining to graph-drawing will only be briefly outlined here.

For the purpose of physiotherapy research the frequency distribution graph is probably the most important. A frequency distribution refers to how *often* a particular event occurs; for instance, how many coronary patients in a particular age group have heart rates of the order of

60–65 beats per minute
66–70 beats per minute
71–75 beats per minute.

The two most common forms of frequency distribution graph are the **histogram** (and related **bar graphs**) and the **frequency polygon**. The features of each will be outlined shortly, but first, we'll look at some points which apply when constructing *all* graphs.

1. It is usual to represent categories of event along the horizontal axis (in the above example, categories of heart rate) and the frequency of their occurrence along the vertical axis. Thus, if you were looking at the vital capacity of cystic fibrosis patients, you would represent the units of vital capacity along the horizontal axis, and the number of patients who showed each vital capacity along the vertical axis:

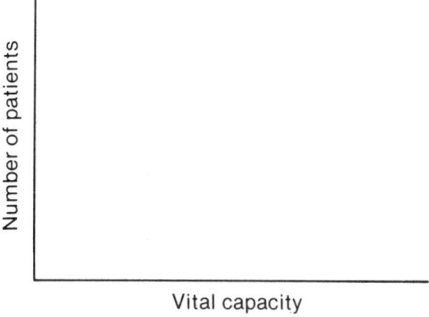

Fig. 2

From this you could see the most common vital capacity score, the range of scores etc. Each axis, as well as the whole graph, should be clearly labelled, such that the graph is self-explanatory.

2. The intersection point of the two axes should represent zero, by convention. If it is more appropriate to alter this to suit your data, make sure this is clear to the reader.

3. Small graphs are hard to construct accurately and equally hard to interpret, so ensure your graph is of reasonable size and that the intervals along the axes are appropriate.

Histograms and bar graphs

These two graphical techniques are very similar, though many people feel the bar graph is clearer. Each technique presents the data in a series of vertical rectangles, with each rectangle representing the number of scores in a particular category. However, with the histogram, the vertical bars are directly adjacent to one another, whereas with the bar graph there are spaces between them. These techniques can best be demonstrated by illustrations. Suppose you want to find out what the social class distribution of multiple sclerosis (MS) sufferers was within your particular region, you might come up with the following figures:

Social class	No. of MS patients
1	15
2	32
3	26
4	10
5	6

These frequencies can be represented either as a histogram or as a bar graph thus:

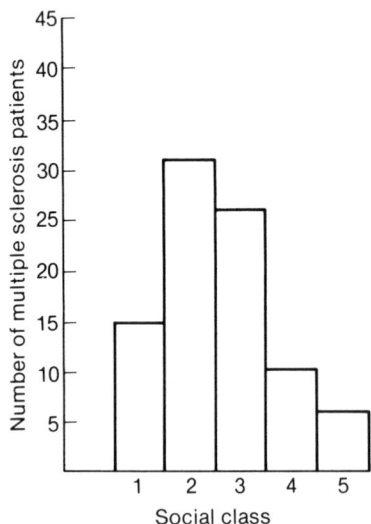

Fig. 3 Histogram showing social class distribution of MS sufferers within a particular region.

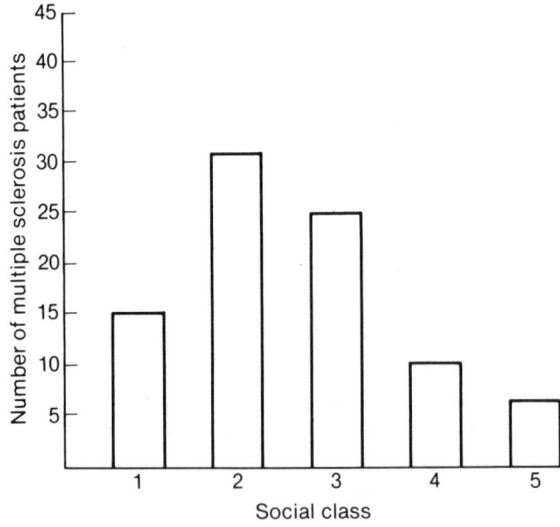

Fig. 4 Bar graph showing social class distribution of MS sufferers within a particular region.

If the categories along the horizontal axis have no natural order, then they may be arranged in order of size, with the greatest frequency distribution on the left and the smallest on the right thus:

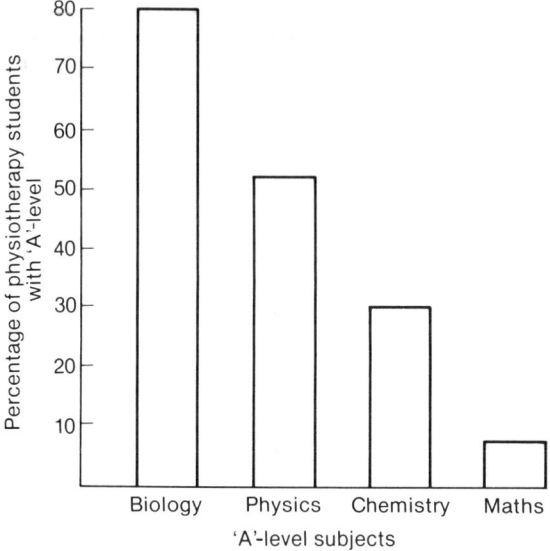

Fig. 5 Bar graph showing comparative frequency of 'A' level subjects among physiotherapy students.

Frequency polygon

The data relating to social class and multiple sclerosis patients could also be plotted as a frequency polygon, in which the frequency of occurrence of each unit or event on the horizontal axis is plotted at the midpoint of the unit, and these points are then joined by a continuous straight line thus:

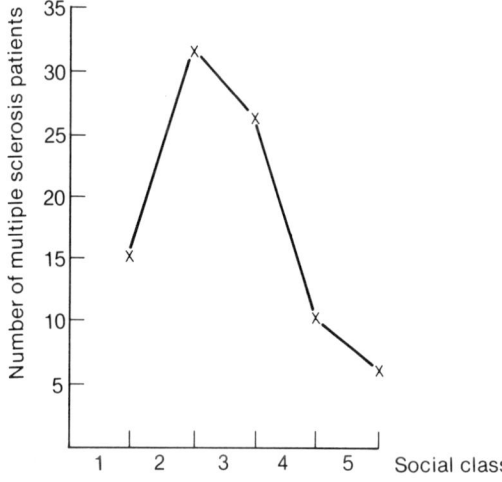

Fig. 6 Frequency polygon showing social class distribution of MS sufferers within a particular region.

In the above example the graph does not touch the horizontal axis. Some people are of the opinion that this gives a rather odd appearance to the graph, and so, in cases where it is appropriate, you can add a class to either end of the units with scores on the horizontal axis. Thus, to give an example you might wish to plot the frequency of average final examination marks across a number of schools of physiotherapy for 1985. The results you obtain are:

Average final exam. mark	No. of schools attaining mark
31–40	0
41–50	1
51–60	3
61–70	4
71–80	1
81–90	1
91–100	0

Your graph might look like this:

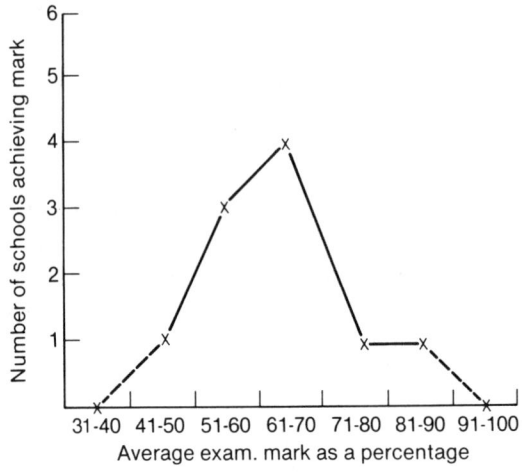

Fig. 7 Frequency polygon showing distribution of average final examination marks across a number of schools of physiotherapy for 1985.

There are *no* schools who achieve an average mark of 31–40% or of 91–100%. Therefore, to give this graph a more complete appearance, the line can be extended to the 0 value for the categories 31–40% and 91–100% (dotted line in Fig. 7).

Obviously, more than one set of data can be plotted on a frequency polygon, so that direct comparisons can be made. In the above example, you might want to plot the average marks for the year 1984 as well, so that you can compare performance.

Whether you decide to use a histogram, bar graph or a frequency polygon depends on the nature of the data you wish to present. Generally, the frequency polygon is more suitable if two or more sets of frequencies are to be compared, since a number of lines can be represented in different colours or styles on the same graph. A similar comparison using bar graphs or histograms is very confusing, since it will involve overlapping rectangles. However, that being said, lay people often find histograms and bar graphs easier to interpret, when they are not familiar with the subject area. In short, which technique you will use will depend on what your objectives are.

There is one further point of interest when plotting frequency distributions. Generally, the larger the amount of data to be plotted, the smoother the resulting frequency distribution curve and conversely, the fewer the scores plotted, the more irregular and uneven the resulting graph. If you are concerned to identify trends, patterns and regularities in your data, you will obviously be keen to produce a smooth frequency distribution. If you cannot achieve this because you have only a limited number of scores to plot, you can obtain greater regularity by reducing the number of categories along the horizontal axis. Let's suppose you were interested in the recovery rates of patients following hysterectomy operations; having looked at some patient records over a 6-month period, you find that:

   4 patients were discharged after 4 days
   6 patients were discharged after 5 days
  10 patients were discharged after 6 days
  13 patients were discharged after 7 days
  10 patients were discharged after 8 days
   9 patients were discharged after 9 days
  15 patients were discharged after 10 days
   3 patients were discharged after 11 days
   5 patients were discharged after 12 days
   2 patients were discharged after 13 days

If this data is plotted as it is presented, we get the following graph:

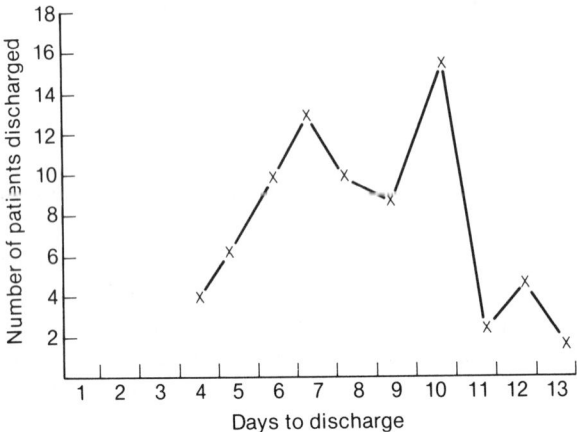

Fig. 8 Frequency polygon showing frequency distribution of recovery period following hysterectomy.

However, if we collapse the categories along the horizontal axis in the following way, we achieve a rather smoother graph:

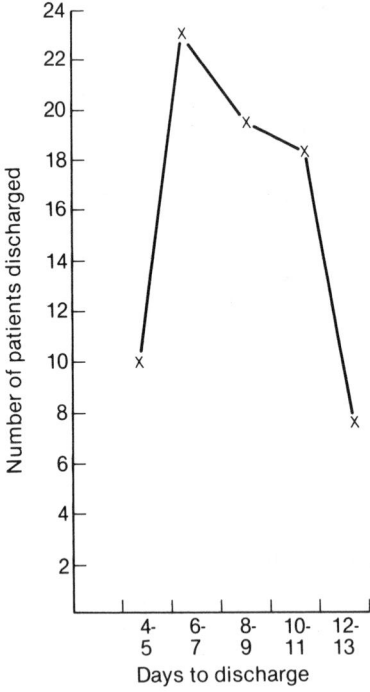

Fig. 9 Frequency polygon showing frequency distribution of recovery period following hysterectomy.

You can see from the above illustration that reducing the categories along the horizontal axis makes the graph appear more regular, and in so doing allows you to get a clearer idea of the trends in the data. (A word of caution, though! Reducing the categories in this way may also distort your data, and obscure important features.)

Shapes of frequency distribution curves

If you plot a large number of graphs over a period of time, you will notice that some shapes of frequency distribution tend to occur time and again. It may be useful to outline some of these briefly.

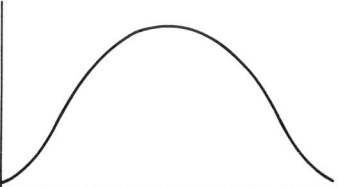

Fig. 10 Normal distribution.

This is probably the most important frequency distribution shape of all and has numerous implications for statistics. So important is it that the next section will be devoted entirely to a more detailed description of it. Suffice it to say for the time being that it is typically a symmetrical bell-shaped curve, and were we to plot heights or heart-rates of a population in this way, we would find that both are normally distributed.

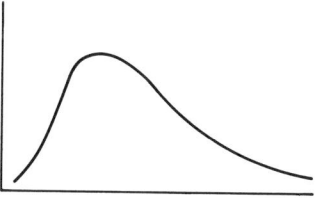

Fig. 11 Skewed distribution (1) — also known as a positive skew.

This frequency distribution is skewed to the left and is the sort of graph that might result from an overly difficult exam, i.e. too many students achieved marks near the bottom end of the score range.

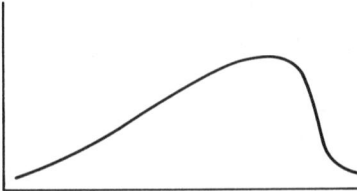

Fig. 12 Skewed distribution (2) — also known as a negative skew.

This graph is skewed in the opposite direction and might have been derived from a set of results from an exam that was too easy.

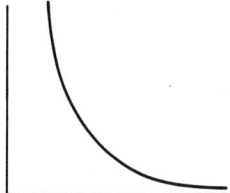

Fig. 13 J-shaped distribution.

This is the sort of frequency distribution which might result from monitoring the number of gastric contractions in a group of patients over a period following a meal. The vast majority of patients would show very few contractions since they would presumably be satisfied; they are represented by the highest part of the graph on the left. However a few people would show rather more activity and they are represented by the flattened tail of the graph to the right.

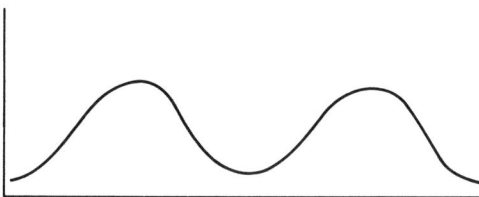

Fig. 14 Bimodal distribution.

This distribution is characterised by two distinct peaks and might have been obtained by plotting the vital capacities of a mixed group of smokers and non-smokers. The smokers would presumably be more likely to have smaller vital capacities and so would be represented by the left-hand peak, while the non-smokers, with larger vital capacities would be represented by the right-hand peak.

Activity 2 (Answers on pages 271–273)

In order to look at the consistency of measurements taken on a goniometer, you ask 15 physiotherapists to measure the knee joint mobility of a post-fracture patient. You obtain the following results:

Degree of movement	No. of physiotherapists recording a particular score
11–20	0
21–30	1
31–40	3
41–50	5
51–60	4
61–70	1
71–80	1
81–90	0

1. Draw (a) a histogram, (b) a bar graph and (c) a frequency polygon to show these results.
2. In order to identify trends in the results, reduce the units along the horizontal axis and re-draw the frequency polygon.

Measures of central tendency

As has already been stated, any results from a piece of research must be presented in a way that can be clearly understood by the reader. Besides making tables of the results and drawing graphs, the data can be presented in terms of *measures of central tendency*.

Measures of central tendency involve describing a set of data in terms of the most typical scores within it. This approach may be valuable to the physiotherapist in three ways:

1. A comparison of some capacity of a group of patients with an established norm or standard for that capacity. For instance you may wish to compare the mobility of a group of hip replacement patients with the normal or average mobility of people of a comparable age group *without* hip trouble.
2. Establishing a standard or norm not previously known, e.g. if a new piece of equipment was introduced to stimulate muscle contraction which you thought may be useful for patients with muscular dystrophy, you would need to establish the level of stimulation provoked in normal muscles by the apparatus as well as in patients' muscles in order to establish what could *normally* be expected from this piece of equipment.
3. Comparing different treatment techniques or different groups of patients, e.g. is clapping more effective than breathing exercises in increasing the vital capacity of cystic fibrosis patients?

In order to answer the questions three measures of central tendency can be used — *the arithmetic mean, the median and the mode.*

Arithmetic mean

This is the average of a set of scores and is derived from adding all the scores together and dividing the total by the number of scores. It is usually denoted by the symbol $\bar{x}$. It is an extremely valuable concept in statistics and enables the researcher to appraise a set of results, at a glance.

For example, in the illustrations given above, the *mean* mobility for the hip-patient group can be compared with the *mean* mobility for the non-patient group to see if there are any overall differences. Similarly, the *mean* vital capacity of the cystic fibrosis patients undergoing breathing exercises can be compared with the *mean* of those undergoing clapping, to give an estimate of which is more effective.

While the arithmetic mean is undoubtedly one of the most useful concepts in statistics, it can be misleading. Supposing you had the choice of giving a frozen shoulder patient one of two treatments. In order to help you make your choice, you turn to some statistics and find that Treatment A produces an average 40% range of movement within 4 weeks, while Treatment B produce 51% range of movement in the same period. From this information alone you would almost certainly favour Treatment B. But let us suppose you were to look at the original data and found the following:

Treatment A		Treatment B	
1.	38%	1.	30%
2.	42%	2.	28%
3.	45%	3.	100%
4.	36%	4.	100%
5.	40%	5.	31%
6.	39%	6.	33%
7.	44%	7.	30%
8.	46%	8.	28%
9.	34%	9.	30%
10.	36%	10.	100%
$\bar{x} =$	40%	$\bar{x} =$	51%

Although Treatment A certainly produces, on average, less range of movement, the results are much more consistent than those from Treatment B; furthermore, with the exception of the three 100% scores, the remaining results in Treatment B are lower than *all* the scores in Treatment A. In other words, the presence of three extreme scores in Treatment B has distorted the means, and could have been misleading had you not looked at the original data. Having examined the raw data, you would probably now choose Treatment A. So, the arithmetic mean, while an essential component to statistics, is insufficient in itself to provide the necessary information about a set of results. Other forms of descriptive statistics are required as well.

Median

The median is simply the mid-score in a set of results, such that there are as many scores above it as below it. To compute the median, arrange the scores in order of magnitude; then if there is an odd number of scores, the middle score becomes the median. So, for example, if you had 5 scores

14   9   28   5   11

you would arrange them in order of magnitude

28   14   11   9   5

and the median becomes the third score from the end, i.e. 11. On the other hand, if there is an even number of scores, the median is the average of the two middle scores. So, if you had

14   9   28   5   11   18

you would arrange these in order of magnitude:

28   18   14   11   9   5

and the median is the average of the two middle scores, i.e. $\dfrac{14 + 11}{2} = 12.5$

While the median obviously tells you the middle score out of a set of results, it tells you nothing about the range of the scores. For example, in the following sets of scores, the median in both cases is 10:

| 13 | 12 | 11 | 10 | 9 | 8 | 7 |
| 99 | 98 | 97 | 10 | 3 | 2 | 1 |

but the nature of the sets of scores is quite different and the *pattern* of a set of scores may have important implications for their interpretation. For instance, if the first set of figures above referred to the ages of patients brought in with a particular disease, you may well think that the disease is age-related. You would not be inclined to think this if presented with the second set of figures. Thus, the nature of the scores is important in research, if they are to be accurately interpreted. So, the median alone gives insufficient information about the nature of a set of data. If it is used in conjunction with the mean, then more information can be derived about the total set of scores. For example, the more similar the mean and median, the smaller the range of scores. This can be illustrated with the above sets of figures. The first set has a mean and a median of 10 and the scores are all within a small range (13–7); however, the second set of figures also has a median of 10 but a mean of 44.3 and a range of scores from 99–1.

While not as useful as the mean, the median is more valuable in describing a set of data where there are very extreme scores.

Mode

The mode is the most commonly occurring score in a set of data. So, in the following two sets of scores, 15 is the mode:

| 15 | 15 | 14 | 10 | 15 | 18 | 15 |
| 15 | 15 | 3 | 2 | 1 | 4 | 5 |

However, within any set of scores, you may have more than one mode. Its value lies primarily in its ability to answer the question 'Which *one* event occurs most often?'. So, for example, you might want to ask which type of cancer occurs most often among women. To do this you simply find out which cancer happens most frequently (i.e. your *modal* score) and you have your answer.

A comparison of the mean, mode and median

Comparing the value of the arithmetic mean, the median and the mode, the mean is the most commonly used statistic and provides more information about a set of scores than the median and the mode. This is due to the fact that the computation of the mean depends on the *exact* value of *every* score in a set of data and alteration of even one score will alter the mean. This is not necessarily the case for the median and the mode as illustrated by the following set of data:

| 3 | 14 | 10 | 19 | 8 | 5 | 15 | 20 | 3 |

The mean of this data is 10.8, the median is 10, and the mode is 3. If we alter the 20 to 40, the mean becomes 13, but the median and the mode stay the same.

In addition, the median and the mode may be totally unaffected by altering a large number of scores in a set of data. If the above set of figures is changed to:

| 3 | 34 | 10 | 39 | 2 | 1 | 45 | 17 | 3 |

although 6 out of 9 figures have been radically altered, the median remains 10 and the mode 3. Conversely, the median and the mode may be *drastically* altered just by the change of one figure. To take the above set of figures, if the first 3 is changed to 34, the median becomes 17 and the mode 34. In other words the median and the mode are less reliable than the mean when providing information about a set of scores because they may not be altered by radical changes to a lot of scores or they may be changed by altering just one score. The mean on the other hand will alter if *any* score is changed, however minimally.

However, as already pointed out, the mean may be less useful than the median or mode if there are extreme scores in a set of data, because it is easily distorted by the presence of very large or small scores. However, although all three concepts can be used in descriptive statistics to provide information about a set of data, it is advisable *always* to calculate the mean, and then to decide whether the median and the mode will provide you with relevant information about your particular set of data.

Key concepts

Measures of central tendency are a form of descriptive statistics and allow the researcher to highlight features of a set of results in terms of the 'most typical values'. The three most commonly used measures of central tendency are:

- the arithmetic mean — the average of a set of scores
- the median — the mid score in a set of results, such that there are as many scores above it as below
- the mode — the most commonly occurring score in a set of data.

Activity 3 (Answers on page 273)

1. Calculate the mean, median and the mode for the following sets of figures:

(i)	91	87	90	76	51	48	72	76	80	44	89	40
(ii)	25	39	17	41	24	17	37	31	27			
(iii)	44	43	51	54	60	71	39	41	55	43		

2. Just by comparing the means and the medians, find out which set of data has (a) the largest range and (b) the smallest range of scores.

Measures of dispersion

If you look back at the measures of central tendency, you will see that it is possible to obtain the same or very similar means for sets of scores which are quite different. For instance, the mean of the following two sets of figures is 10:

9	11	12	8	10	11	12	12	8	7
1	2	3	3	2	1	40	3	15	30

However, the scores in the first set are all quite similar to each other in that they only range from 7 to 12; the scores in the second set, however, range from 1 to 40. Just knowing the *mean* of a set of scores, then, can be quite misleading — we need to know how *variable* the socres are as well, in other words, what the spread of the data is. The statistics which describe the variability of scores are called *measures of dispersion* and are valuable to the physiotherapist for the same reasons as the measures of central tendency. If you look back to page 21, you will see that the first reason given is that the researcher can compare a group of patients with an established standard to discover how far their capacity, mobility, skills or whatever resemble the norm. This can be carried out just using means, medians, and modes, but we have already seen that similar means can be obtained from two totally different sets of scores. So, if we use the example on page 21, you might find that 4 out of 5 of your hip relacement patients had extremely limited mobility, while one had much greater mobility than the non-patient group. If you simply combine the mobility scores of these 5 patients and take the mean you may well find that due to the one very mobile patient, the mean is very similar to that of the non-patient group — and yet 4 of the patients were barely mobile. In other words you need to know what the *spread* of scores is. Similarly if you wish to establish norms for a new piece of apparatus, it is insufficient just to use measures of central tendency, because they can be misleading unless you know how consistent the scores are. Obviously a piece of equipment which produces uniformly good results will be much more use than one which produces an entire range of results from poor to excellent even though the mean performances may be similar. In addition, measures of dispersion can identify patients who respond particularly well or particularly poorly. This information may be useful when selecting treatments. And similarly, when comparing two or more treatment types, the treatment which produces homogeneous results, i.e. where the range of scores is small, will be regarded quite differently from the treatment which produces erratic results which cover an enormous range. So, in descriptive statistics, not only do you need to use measures of central tendency, you also need to describe the results in terms of how variable they are and to do this you use techniques called measures of dispersion. There are three measures of dispersion which are valuable to the physiotherapist — *the range, deviation and variance and the standard deviation.*

Range

The range is quite simply the difference between lowest and highest scores in a set of data. To compute it, simply find the smallest score in the data and subtract it from the highest score, thus:

| 14 | 22 | 5 | 11 | 12 | 19 | 31 | 27 |

the range is $31 - 5 = 26$

Obviously, when used in conjunction with measures of central tendency, it can provide useful additional information, in the way already outlined. However, the information produced by the range gives a limited picture since a range of 45–3 may describe a set of scores such as:

| 45 | 44 | 43 | 42 | 7 | 6 | 5 | 4 | 3 |

or

| 45 | 40 | 35 | 30 | 30 | 15 | 10 | 5 | 3 |

In other words, the range provides no insight into *how the scores are distributed*. One way of getting round this problem is to use *deviation and variance measures.*

Deviation and variance

One method of overcoming the problem of presenting a picture of the distribution of scores is by expressing the scores in terms of how far each one *deviates* from the mean. In this way the researcher can present a description of the spread of scores, which, as we've seen, is important in understanding the implications of a set of data.

In order to calculate the deviation of a set of scores, the mean is substracted from each score. Thus, for the following set of scores:

10   15   21   8   11   12   14   5

the mean is 12 and the deviation of each score is:

$$10 - 12 = -2$$
$$15 - 12 = +3$$
$$21 - 12 = +9$$
$$8 - 12 = -4$$
$$11 - 12 = -1$$
$$12 - 12 = 0$$
$$14 - 12 = +2$$
$$5 - 12 = -7$$

In subtracting the mean from each score, you can find the position of each score relative to the mean. So, for example, the score of 15 is $+3$ deviation points above the mean.

However, as you can probably see, expressing each score as a deviation from the mean is just as long-winded as setting out all your scores and their means — what is needed is some short-hand method of expressing how varied and dispersed the scores are. While many students assume that the obvious way would be to add together all the deviation scores, the answer is always 0 (try it for yourself and see) so this clearly tells us nothing. So, one way of getting round this problem is to *square* each deviation score (this obviously gets rid of all the plus and minus signs) and then to add these squared deviation scores up. The total is called the *variance*.

If we compute the variance for the set of scores above, we get:

$$(-2^2) + (3^2) + (9^2) + (-4^2) + (-1^2) + (0^2) + (2^2) + (-7^2)$$
$$= 4 + 9 + 81 + 16 + 1 + 0 + 4 + 49$$
$$= 164$$

The variance of a set of scores tells us by definition how dispersed or varied the scores are. Obviously, the smaller the variance, the more similar the scores, while the greater the variance the more disparate the scores. If you look back to the example on page 22 about the frozen shoulder treatments, you can see that knowledge of the spread of scores would be a very useful piece of information here, since the *smaller* the variance the more reliable and consistent the treatment procedure.

Standard deviation

Although the variance score gives you the total degree of variability in a set of scores, it has been obtained, obviously, by adding together such varied squared deviations as 81 and 0 (see the previous set of figures). Sometimes you may want to find out what the average or *standard* degree of deviation is for a set of scores, rather than the *total* degree of variation. To do this you need a very useful statistic called, not unreasonably, the standard deviation (or SD).

To calculate it, you simply take the variance figure (i.e. the total of the squared deviation scores — in the above case, 164), divide this by the total number of scores (to give the average squared deviation) and then take the square root of this, to give you the standard deviation of the scores from the mean.

The formula then is:

$$SD = \sqrt{\frac{\Sigma(x - \bar{x})^2}{N}}$$

where $\sqrt{}$ = square root of all the calculations under this symbol
x = the individual score
$\bar{x}$ = the mean score
Σ = total, or sum, of every calculation to the right
N = the total number of scores.

(You may have realised that $\Sigma(x - \bar{x})^2$ is the variance score.)
So, for the figures above, the standard deviation is

$$\sqrt{\frac{164}{8}}$$
$$= 4.528$$

Sometimes you will find the SD formula given as $\sqrt{\dfrac{\Sigma(x - \bar{x})^2}{N - 1}}$

The $N - 1$ is used if you want to *infer* the standard deviation of the population from which your sample is drawn, whereas just N describes the standard deviation of the sample *only*. However, in practice, this variation makes very little difference, so don't worry unduly about it.

This means that the standard degree of deviation of this set of scores from the mean is 4.528. Such information gives you a picture of how dispersed or variable a set of scores is in a single figure — which as we've already pointed out is particularly useful in determining the consistency of a set of figures.

All of this may seem rather confusing to you when deciding how to describe a set of data. As a rule of thumb, I would recommend that you always calculate the mean, range and standard deviation of a set of scores and then decide which of the other measures provides you with information which is relevant to the aims of that particular piece of research.

> **Key concept**
>
> Measures of dispersion are a branch of descriptive statistics which allow the researcher to describe a set of data in terms of how variable the scores are.
>
> The three measures of dispersion which are of particular importance to the physiotherapist are:
>
> - the range — the difference between the lowest and highest score in a set of data
> - the deviation — provides information about the extent *each* score deviates from the mean, and is expressed as a plus or minus figure for each score.
> - the variance — the total amount that a *set* of scores deviates from the mean and is calculated by squaring each deviation score and adding the results up.
>
> The standard deviation (SD) is the average amount of deviation and is computed by dividing the variance by the total number of scores and taking the square root of this result.

Activity 4 (Answers on pages 273–274)

1. Find the range, deviation, variance and standard deviation of the following sets of scores:

   (i) 14   9   21   23   18   17   33   28   12
   (ii) 71   50   48   64   80   81   79
2. You are concerned about one of the goniometers in use in your department, since you are not sure how reliable it is. How might you assess its reliability using descriptive statistics?

Normal distribution

It was pointed out earlier that there are a number of frequency distribution shapes which occur commonly in statistics. The most common of all these is the so-called *normal distribution curve* (sometimes know as the Gaussian distribution, after Gauss, the astronomer and mathematician who investigated it). The normal distribution curve is a symmetrical bell-shaped distribution:

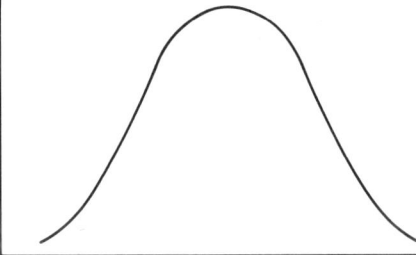

Fig. 15 Normal distribution curve

It possesses a number of important mathematical properties:

a. It is symmetrical.
b. The mean, median and mode all have the same value.
c. The curve descends rapidly at first from its central point, but the descent slows down as the tails of the curve are reached.
d. No matter how far you continue the tails of the curve, they never reach the horizontal axis.
e. The normal distribution curve occurs in data drawn from a wide range of subjects — mathematics, physics, engineering, psychology etc. For example, height, IQ and the life of electric light bulbs all have normal distributions. In other words, if we collected, for example, height data from a large number of people randomly drawn from the population and drew a frequency distribution of it, we would end up with something that resembled a normal curve.
f. If the mean and standard deviation of a normally distributed set of data are known, then we can draw the normal distribution curve. The reason this can be done results from the relationship between the standard deviation and the normal distribution curve. This relationship means that a fixed percentage of the scores always falls in a given area under the curve. Therefore, if we take the central point of the curve:

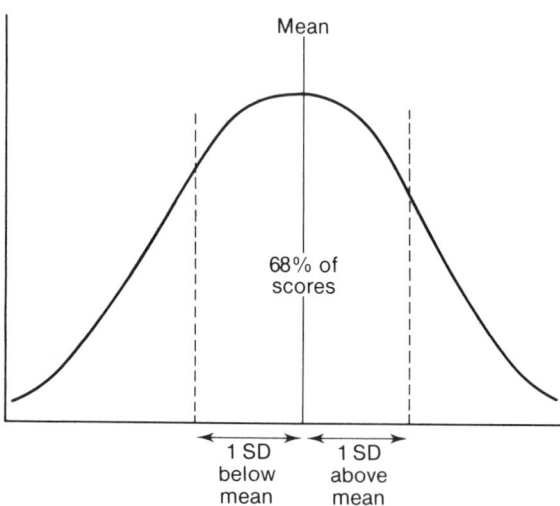

Fig. 16

and then move one standard deviation above and below the mean, then 68% of the scores will *always* fall within this range. This is a constant fact of the normal distribution, i.e. that 34% of scores fall within one standard deviation *above* the mean, and 34% of scores fall one standard deviation *below*.

If we move on, we find that a further 13.5% of the scores fall between standard deviations 1 and 2 *above* the mean, and 13.5% fall between standard deviations 1 and 2 *below* the mean. Thus, the two standard deviations either side of the mean account for a total of 95% of the scores (13.5 + 34 + 34 + 13.5). Going on to standard deviations 2–3 above and below the mean, we find that 2.36% of scores fall within each category, thereby allowing a total of 99.73% of the scores to be accounted for by 3 standard deviations above and below the mean (2.36 + 13.5 + 34 + 34 + 13.5 + 2.36 = 99.72, represented normally as 99.73 as a result of further decimal places).

So, to take an example, if we know that the mean IQ of the population is 100 and the standard deviation is 20, then 68% of the population have IQs between 80 and 120, 95% have IQs between 60 and 140, and 99.73% have IQs between 40 and 160. We can see this more clearly in the normal curve below:

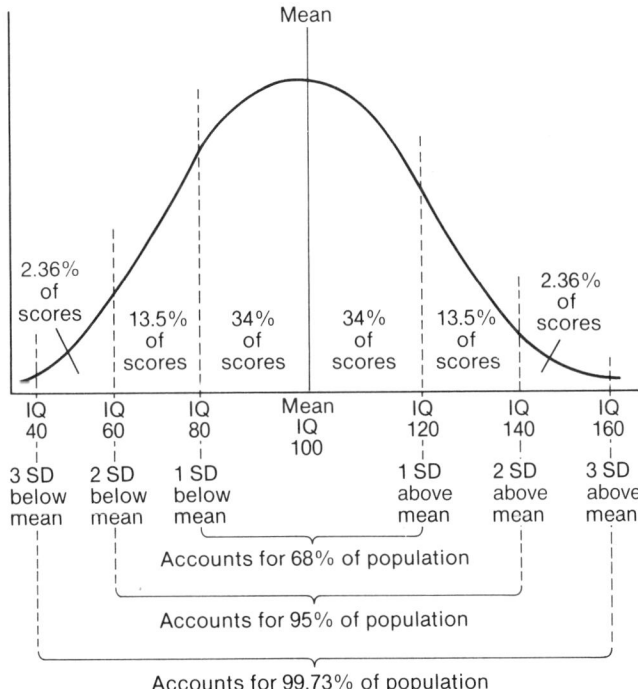

Fig. 17 Hypothetical normal distribution curve for IQ

The value of the normal distribution is twofold. Firstly, it allows the researcher to describe a set of data and to predict (from knowledge of the properties of the normal curve) what proportions of people possess certain characteristics.

For example, if we know that the *average* heart rate is 72, with a standard deviation of 5, and that heart rate is normally distributed, we can draw the curve:

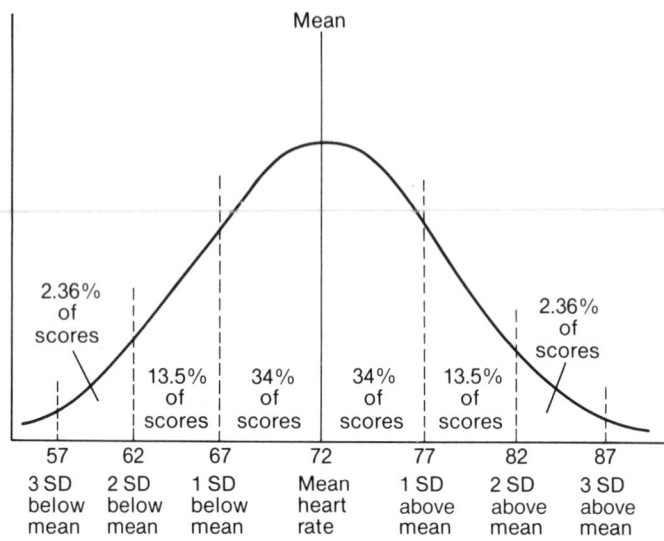

Fig. 18 Hypothetical normal distribution curve for heart rate

Now, because we know that 68% of people are accounted for by scores within 1 standard deviation either side of the mean, we know that 68% of the population must have heart rates between 67 and 77 beats per minute. Furthermore, we know a further 13.5% of people fall within standard deviations 1 and 2 above the mean and a further 13.5% fall within standard deviations 1 and 2 below the mean. This means 13.5% of the population have heart rates of 77–82 beats per minute and 13.5% have heart rates of 62–67 beats per minute. Finally, we know that 2.36% of the population fall within standard deviations 2–3 above the mean and a further 2.36% within standard deviations 2–3 below the mean. This means 2.36% of people have heart rates of 82–87 beats per minute and 2.36% have heart rates of 57–62 beats per minute. This information also allows us to 'work backwards'; if a patient presents with a heart rate of 86, then you can ascertain just how statistically unusual this is, since you know that only 2.36% of the population come within this range.

The second function of the normal distribution curve relates to its role in inferential statistics. Many of the tests used in inferential statistics require that the results being analysed are normally distributed (see section on *parametric* statistics); if they are not, then these tests are inappropriate and other sorts of test (i.e. *non*-parametric tests) must be used. This will be explained in more detail in Chapter 6. The normal distribution curve also underlies some of the theoretical assumptions of inferential statistics, although these need not concern us unduly here.

Key concepts

The normal distribution curve is a commonly occurring frequency distribution which possesses certain mathematical properties:

- if the mean and the standard deviation of set of scores are known, then the researcher is able to predict what proportion of the population have scores within a certain range. This is possible because a fixed proportion of the population will fall within a certain score range, as long as those scores are normally distributed.
- the normal curve is of fundamental importance in the theory behind inferential statistics.

Activity 5 (Answers on page 274)

1. If we know that heart rate during weeks 10–20 of pregnancy is normally distributed, with a mean of 82 and a standard deviation of 8, then:

   (i) What percentage of patients will have heart rates between 66 and 98
   (ii) What percentage of patients will show heart rates of 99–106
   (iii) If a patient presents with a heart rate of 57, how common is this in terms of percentage?

3

Inferential statistics: some basic concepts involved in designing research projects which test a specific hypothesis

We have just briefly covered the topic of descriptive statistics, which provide the researcher with one method of presenting data. However, this approach is typically used to make sense of data derived from some form of survey and is not appropriate for analysing results from an *experiment*, where an hypothesis has been tested. What is needed here, is a second branch of statistics known as *inferential statistics*.

There will be many occasions when you do not want simply to collect a mound of general information about a broad topic area, but wish, instead, to test out an idea, for instance, comparing the effectiveness of two treatment techniques, or monitoring the progress of a specific group of patients. In such cases, you would analyse the results from this using a statistical test. This sort of analysis is called *inferential statistics*, and is so-called because it allows you to *infer* that the results you obtained from your experiment using a small sample of people may also apply to the larger population from which the sample was drawn. Look back to pages 10–12 to refresh your memory on this.

However, before you can reasonably start inferring anything from the results of an experiment, it is essential that the experiment is properly set up and designed, otherwise *false* inferences may be made. This chapter and the next are concerned with outlining the principles of good experimental techniques.

When carrying out any research which involves testing an hypothesis, the following steps have to be taken:

— an hypothesis must be devised and stated clearly
— a research project must be designed which will test the hypothesis
— results from the research have to be analysed using an appropriate statistical test
— a report must be prepared on the research for future reference.

We shall deal with each of these stages in turn. The present chapter will be concerned with the principles involved in devising hypotheses and some basic concepts about research design.

EXPERIMENTAL HYPOTHESIS

The starting point of any research is an idea known as the *experimental or research hypothesis* — sometimes referred to as H_1. This is usually based on some theory or observations that the potential experimenter has made. You may, for instance, have noticed in the course of your work, that certain patients seem to respond better to particular types of treatment. An observation of this type would form the basis of an experimental hypothesis. Examples of experimental hypotheses include such ideas as the following:

1. Male physiotherapy students perform better in clinical assessment than female physiotherapy students.
2. Leg fracture patients make quicker recoveries with traction than with cast-bracing.
3. Job satisfaction is greater among community physiotherapists than hospital-based physiotherapists.

You probably have a number of such ideas that you are interested in looking at, and it would be useful to write them down at this stage.

If we look at the above hypotheses, we can see that what the experimental hypothesis does is to *predict a relationship* between two or more things, known as *variables**. Therefore, the first hypothesis predicts a relationship between *sex* of the physiotherapy student (male or female), and *performance* in clinical assessments. The two variables here, then, are sex of student and performance. The second hypothesis predicts a relationship between *type of treatment* (traction or cast bracing), and *speed of recovery*. The two variables here are type of treatment and recovery rate. The third hypothesis predicts a relationship between *degree of job satisfaction* and *type of physiotherapist* (community or hospital). The two variables, then, are job satisfaction and type of physiotherapist.

Key concept

The experimental hypothesis is the starting point of any research and predicts a relationship between two or more variables.

Activity 6 (Answers on page 274)

Look at the following hypotheses and write down what the two variables are in each case.

1. Children with leg fractures progress faster on traction than adoloscents with leg fractures.

---

* Throughout the course of this book, we shall deal with hypotheses and experiments that predict a relationship between only *two* variables. If the reader wants to find out about hypotheses which deal with a predicted relationship between *more* than two variables then the following books are recommended: Greene & D'Oliviera (1982) and Ferguson (1976).

2. Men and women with arthritis differ in their responsiveness to heat treatment.
3. Men are more likely to suffer chest infections following cardiothoracic surgery than are women.
4. Outpatients' clinics achieve better recovery rates for leg fractures than specific sports injuries clinics.
5. There is a difference in professional competence between physiotherapists who trained in hospital-based training schools than those who trained in polytechnic-based training schools.

Now think about the research project you would like to carry out. State the experimental hypothesis, making sure it predicts a relationship between the two variables. Write down what the variables are.

Now in order to find out whether the relationship predicted in your hypothesis does, in fact, exist, you have to proceed to the next stage and design and carry out a suitable project to test your hypothesis. Any results you get from the research are then analysed using the appropriate statistical test. But, before we move on to talk about how you proceed, one very important point must be made.

NULL HYPOTHESIS

It must be logically possible for the relationship predicted in your experimental hypothesis to be wrong, otherwise there is no point in wasting your time carrying out any research. For example, anyone who hypothesised that all physiotherapists who were born in 1940 are older than those born in 1945 and then spent 3 days amongst the record books trying to support their hypothesis would be indulging in a pointless exercise, since there would be absolutely no possibility that their prediction would be wrong. Therefore, to make any research project worthwhile, there has to be a chance that the predicted relationship does *not* exist. To show that there is a possibility that the experimental hypothesis is incorrect, we have to state an alternative hypothesis called the *null hypothesis*. This is sometimes referred to as H_0. So, while the experimental hypothesis predicts that there *is* a relationship between two variables, the null hypothesis says there is *no* relationship and that any results you get from your research project are due to chance and *not* to any real and significant relationship between the variables. Let's take an example. Supposing in the course of your work you have noticed that Asian patients are more likely to follow oral instructions for exercises following leg fractures than written instructions. You decide to carry out some research to see if your hunch is right. The first step is to state the experimental hypothesis clearly, i.e. 'Asian patients are more likely to comply with oral exercise instructions than written exercise instructions following leg fractures.' So, you are predicting a relationship between the type of instructions given and degree of compliance. But because it is possible that your observations are wrong, you must also state the null hypothesis that there is *no* relationship between the type of instructions and degree of compliance. The null hypothesis also implies that any differences in degree of compliance that you find in your results are simply due to chance fluctuations and not to any real and consistent relationship. The usual way of stating the null hypothesis is simply to predict *no* relationship between the two variables. Therefore, here, your null hypothesis would be: 'There is no relationship between type of instructions and degree of compliance.'

If you ever get stuck when formulating the null hypothesis, the easy way to get round the problem is by:

a. firstly identifying the relationship in the experimental hypothesis, by stating 'There is a relationship between a and b.'
b. changing the first part to 'There is no relationship between . . . .' This gives you your null hypothesis.

It is very important to note that the null hypothesis predicts **no** relationship; it does *not* predict the opposite of the experimental hypothesis. Many students get confused over this and in the example just given would assume that the null hypothesis says the reverse of the experimental hypothesis — that written instructions are more likely to be followed than oral ones. (Just refresh your memory and check that this is the opposite of our original hypothesis.) This assumption is incorrect, because if we look at it, a relationship is *still* being predicted between type of instructions and compliance. So, the null hypothesis says there is *no* relationship between the two variables — in this case type of instruction and degree of compliance.

Activity 7 (Answers on pages 274–275)

To see whether you are happy with this concept, look at the experimental hypotheses on pages 36–37 and write down what the null hypothesis is for each one. State the null hypothesis for the research project you would like to carry out.

Why do we need to state the null hypothesis at all? Could we not just assume that there is a chance that our experimental hypothesis may be wrong without having to spell it out? The answer to this lies in a convention, which has its roots in the philosophy of scientific method (for further details on this the reader is referred to Chalmers (1983)).

Essentially this convention states that when we carry out any research we do not set out to find direct support for our experimental hypothesis (or at least we shouldn't!) but, rather perversely, to *falsify the null hypothesis*. In other words we still hope to find the relationship we predicted in the experimental hypothesis, but we do this by stating the null hypothesis and setting out to reject it. It should be noted here that the words 'prove' and 'disprove' in relation to the hypotheses are not being used. This is because we cannot really ever prove or disprove anything in physiotherapy, psychology or whatever — all we can do is find evidence that supports or fails to support our prediction. The intending researcher need not worry unduly about all this, since it is sufficient simply to state the experimental and null hypotheses at the outset of any experiment. The relevance of the null hypothesis will be discussed further in the chapter on writing up research.

> **Key concepts**
>
> The null hypothesis states that the relationship predicted in the experimental hypothesis does **not** exist and implies that any results found from the research are simply due to chance factors and not to any real and consistent relationship between the two variables. In any research project, the experimenter sets out to support his/her prediction by rejecting the null hypothesis.

BASIC TYPES OF DESIGN

Once you have sorted out the experimental and null hypotheses for your research project, you then have to decide on the best way to find out whether your predicted relationship actually exists. In other words you have to *design a suitable research project*. It should be noted that there are often a *number* of designs that can be used to test an hypothesis, and it is up to the researcher to select the most appropriate one. The concept that there is usually no *single* correct way of testing an hypothesis, means that the researcher must take into account a number of design considerations, and it is with these that this chapter and the following one are concerned.

There are two basic sorts of research designs — *experimental designs* and *correlational designs*. Both designs start off with an experimental hypothesis which predicts a relationship between two or more variables, but the aims and methods of each approach are different. These differences can be best illustrated by an example. Let's take the hypothesis that the professional rank of physiotherapist affects the degree of job satisfaction that is experienced. The relationship that is being suggested is between professional status of the physiotherapist and degree of job satisfaction. Let's see how experimental and correlational designs would each approach the problem of trying to find out whether this relationship does, in fact, exist.

Experimental designs

The experimental design would take a group of senior physiotherapists (say 10 district physiotherapists) and a group of junior physiotherapists (say, physiotherapists), measure the reported job satisfaction expressed by each group and compare the two groups to see if there was any *difference* between them.

We would have the following design:

Group 1
10 district physiotherapists

Group 2
10 physiotherapists

Compared on expressed job satisfaction for *differences* between the groups

Correlational designs

The correlational design, on the other hand, would select a number of physiotherapists who represented the whole *range* of professional status from physiotherapist through to district level and measure their reported job satisfaction to see if there is any *similarity* or *association* between professional level and degree of job satisfaction, such that, for instance, the higher the status, the higher the corresponding job satisfaction.

The correlational design would look like this:

Subject	Level of physiotherapist	Job satisfaction scores (on a 10-point scale)
1	District	9
2	Superintendent I	8
3	Superintendent IV	5
4	Senior	4
5	Physiotherapist	4

Status and job satisfaction would be compared to see if there is any similarity or association between them.

Experimental and correlational designs will be discussed more fully in the next two sections. It should be stressed, however, that for the hypothesis we are looking at, *either* design would be appropriate. This illustrates the idea that was mentioned earlier — that for any hypothesis there may be a number of suitable designs to test it, and it is up to the researcher to think carefully about the aims, objectives and the relevant design considerations of the research and to devise the most appropriate method of testing the hypothesis.

Key concepts

Experimental designs look for *differences* between sets of results. Correlational designs look for *similarities* between sets of results. Therefore, each approach has a different objective and will consequently use a different method to test the hypothesis.

We will deal with the basic principles involved in each design separately, starting with experimental designs.

EXPERIMENTAL DESIGNS

We have already noted that the experimental hypothesis predicts a relationship between two variables. The simplest way to find out whether this relationship actually exists is to alter one of these variables to see what difference it makes to the other. This is the basis of experimental design. This alteration is known as *manipulation of variables*, and is actually something we do in everyday life, often without being aware of it. This can be illustrated by a mundane example. Suppose you were babysitting for a friend and had decided to watch their television. You turn it on and discover that the sound is too low. Because you aren't familiar with the controls on this set you aren't sure how to adjust the volume, but you think it might be the knob on the front of the set. Unwittingly, you have formulated an hypothesis — that there is a relationship between the knob and the volume. In order to test this hypothesis, you have to manipulate one of the variables — in other words, you alter the knob to see what effect it has on the sound. You have just performed a very simple experiment, which involved hypothesising a relationship between two variables and manipulating one to see what difference it made to the other. This is the basis of experimental design.

How do you decide which of the two variables to manipulate? If we look back at the television set example, the answer to this is logical since we cannot possibly manipulate the volume to see what effect it has on the knob! Therefore, if you are ever unsure which of the two variables in your hypothesis has to be manipulated, just think about the effect each has on the other and the answer should be obvious.

These variables have names. The variable which is manipulated is called the *Independent Variable* (IV) and the variable which is observed or measured for any changes or differences is called the *Dependent Variable* (DV) (because it is *dependent* on the manipulation of the other variable). Thus, the IV can be seen as *cause* and the DV as *effect*. Just to illustrate this idea, let's take the hypothesis that leg fractures improve more quickly with traction than with cast bracing. The two variables are type of treatment and speed of recovery. Which variable is which? We obviously cannot manipulate speed of recovery to find out what effect it has on type of treatment, so it must be type of treatment that is manipulated to see whether it made any difference to the speed of recovery. Therefore, type of treatment is the independent variable and speed of recovery is the dependent variable because how quickly a patient recovers *depends* on the treatment received. What is meant here, then, when we talk about manipulating the Independent Variable is simply assigning some patients to traction and some to cast bracing. Their progress is then compared. However, the problem is not always quite as simple as this. Supposing we hypothesised that there is a difference between the responses of male and female patients to ultrasound. Here the dependent variable is the difference in response to ultrasound, so the independent variable must be the sex of the patient. But how does the experimenter manipulate the sex of the patient? Obviously in the previous example, it was easy for the experimenter to decide which treatment a fracture patient should receive, but in the latter case we cannot possibly take a group of patients and decide what sex they should be! In this case the experimenter would simply select two groups of patients, one male and one female, and compare their responses to ultrasound. The independent variable is still being manipulated but in a slightly different way. Obviously, this sort of manipulation is essential when the independent variable is of a 'fixed' nature, such as race, age, type of patient etc.

Activity 8 (Answers on page 275)

Look at the following hypotheses and decide which is the independent variable, and which is the dependent variable. When you have done that, decide how you would manipulate the independent variable. If you find that you are having difficulty deciding which variable is which, just ask yourself which variable *depends* on which.

1. Men and women differ in their tendency to complain about pain.
2. Zimmer frames are more effective than walking sticks in aiding the mobility of arthritis patients.
3. Absenteeism is greater amongst physiotherapists working in psychiatric hospitals than amongst physiotherapists working in general hospitals.
4. Physiotherapists are able to establish greater rapport with male patients than with female patients.
5. Physiotherapy schools who require 'A'-level physics have higher pass rates on CSP exams than schools who do not require 'A'-level physics.

Key concepts

Experimental designs involve manipulating the *Independent Variable* and measuring the effect of this on the *Dependent Variable*. The Independent Variable can be thought of as *cause* and the Dependent Variable as *effect*.

So far we have assumed that all experimental hypotheses have just one independent variable. However, as we mentioned earlier, this is not always the case and some more complex hypotheses and experiments may predict a relationship between two or more independent variables and the dependent variable. An example of this sort of hypothesis would be a predicted relationship between the age of a patient and his/her response to one or more treatment types, e.g. that there is a difference in improvement rate of children and adolescents with cystic fibrosis to clapping or exercise techniques. Here the dependent variable is improvement rate and the independent variables are the age of the patient and the type of treatment they receive. This hypothesis requires a rather more complicated design, which is outside the scope of this book, but the reader is referred to Greene & D'Oliviera (1982) or Ferguson (1976) for more details on experimental designs with more than one independent variable. In this book we shall deal only with experiments which test hypotheses with just one independent variable.

Some basic principles involved in designing experiments with one independent variable

To recap, experimental designs require the experimenter to manipulate or alter the independent variable and to measure the effect of this on the dependent variable. In other words, you alter one variable and measure the *difference* it makes to the other. Hence experimental designs are said to look for differences. It is important to note that this applies only to experimental designs and not to correlational designs which we shall look at in the next section.

. So, having formulated your experimental hypothesis and null hypothesis, the next task is to design a suitable experiment to find out whether the relationship predicted in your hypothesis exists. The basic concepts involved in this are best explained by an example. Suppose you wanted to test the hypothesis that physiotherapists who did a psychology course run by the local college became more tolerant in their attitudes to patients. The independent variable is attendance on a course and the dependent variable is attitude change. To test this hypothesis you decide to give those physiotherapists who have completed a psychology course an attitude questionnaire. Therefore you would have the following design:

Independent variable		*Dependent variable*
Attendance on on course	$\longrightarrow$	Measurement of attitudes

What could you conclude from the replies to the questionnaire? Could you assume that the physiotherapists' attitudes had changed or not? You have probably quite correctly decided that we cannot conclude anything from this study since we don't know what their attitudes were in the first place. So an essential feature of an experiment is a *pre-test measure* of the dependent variable. Let's revise our design to include this:

1. Pre-test measure of DV (attitudes)	2. Attendance on course (IV)	3. Post-test measure of DV (attitudes)

What could you conclude from this experiment now? You could certainly decide on the basis of some statistical analysis of the pre-test and post-test scores whether there had been a significant attitude change but you couldn't ascribe it *necessarily* to course attendance, since it is quite possible that there are other explanations for change.

Activity 9 (Answers on page 275)

Can you think of any possible alternative reasons for these results?

Certainly, it is conceivable that these physiotherapists might have become more tolerant anyway, simply because they were just a bit older, and a bit more experienced. They might also have changed jobs, got promotion or had any one of a number of experiences which might account for their attitude change. How, then, can we ever be sure that the results in our experiment are due to the independent variable? The only way to do this is to select **two** groups of physiotherapists and to make sure that the *only* difference between the groups is whether or not they experience the independent variable. So, going back to our example, we would select two groups of physiotherapists, of which just *one* group had attended a psychology course and we would compare their post-test attitudes. Our revised design looks like this:

Group 1 Physiotherapists who attend a psychology course

Pre-test measure of DV (attitudes)	Attendance on course (IV)	Post-test measure of DV (attitudes)

Group 2 Physiotherapists who have not attended a psychology course

Pre-test measure of DV (attitudes)	No attendance on course (no IV)	Post-test measure of DV (attitudes)

These two groups are given names — the group who receives the independent variable (in this case, attends a psychology course) is called the *Experimental Condition*. The group who does not receive the independent variable (in this case, does not attend a psychology course) is called the *Control Condition*. The variation between the pre-test and post-test scores from the two conditions are compared using a statistical test to find out if there are any significant *differences* between them.

Key concepts

The subjects in the Experimental Condition are subjected to the Independent Variable.
The Control Condition subjects are *not* subjected to the Independent Variable.

There are still many flaws in our design but we will talk about ways of eliminating them and refining an experiment in the next chapter. Nonetheless, the Key Concepts that have been outlined should give you an idea about some of the fundamental issues involved in experimental designs.

By now you might be wanting to raise some moral issues. This sort of design is fine when we want to look at something like the effects of a psychology course on attitudes. In this instance, there is no moral dilemma about *not* giving physiotherapists a psychology course. But supposing your hypothesis was that cystic fibrosis patients would improve significantly on a new exercise regime. The IV here is the treatment and the DV is the improvement. You select your two groups of patients, and you give the experimental group your new treatment, but according to the above principles of experimental design, the other group of cystic fibrosis patients should receive *no* treatment. Is this ethical? Surely we cannot possibly leave a group of patients with no treatment while we are busily testing out our ideas? In cases such as this, you would compare *two* experimental groups rather than *one* experimental group and *one* control group. So, instead of comparing your new treatment with *no* treatment, you would compare it with the conventional treatment or another form of treatment. Our design would look like this:

Experimental Condition 1
Pre-test   New exercise   Post-test measure
measure of DV   regime (IV)   of DV

Experimental Condition 2
Pre-test   Conventional   Post-test measure
measure of DV   treatment (IV)   of DV

In this case, *both* groups are subjected to the Independent Variable (treatment) and their progress compared, to find out whether there are any *differences* between the groups.

Activity 10 (Answers on pages 275–276)
Look at the following hypotheses and set out the experimental design you would use in each case, using the sort of format and headings shown above:
Hypotheses
1. Patients are more relaxed with physiotherapists who wear uniform than with those who do not wear uniform.
2. Physiotherapists who have been a hospital patient are more sympathetic than those who have not.
3. Physiotherapists who have qualified in the last 5 years are more motivated than those who have been qualified for more than 10 years.

The sort of design we have been looking at is the most simple experimental design of all — a pre-test measure of the dependent variable, manipulation of the independent variable and a post-test measure of the dependent variable. Two groups are used, of which one may be a control condition or alternatively, both groups may be experimental conditions. However, you may become a bit more ambitious and decide that you would like to look at something a little more complex than this. If we look back to our last hypothesis — that cystic fibrosis patients make significant improvements on a new exercise regime, we have used a design which involved the comparison of *two* experimental groups. But you could, if you wished, add further conditions to this design. If you managed to resolve any ethical problem in your mind, you might decide to add a control condition as well, and so your design would look like this:

Experimental Condition 1

| Pre-test measure of DV | New exercise regime (IV) | Post-test measure of DV |

Experimental Condition 2

| Pre-test measure of DV | Conventional treatment (IV) | Post-test measure of DV |

Control Condition

| Pre-test measure of DV | No treatment (no IV) | Post-test measure of DV |

So you still have two experimental *conditions, or levels* of the independent variable, but you now have a control condition as well. Alternatively, you might feel that it would be useful to compare three types of therapy instead of two, perhaps adding heat treatment to the exercise regime and conventional therapy. Therefore, your hypothesis would be something like 'exercise, heat treatment and conventional therapy are differentially effective in helping cystic fibrosis patients.' The dependent variable is degree of improvement and the independent variable is still type of treatment, but this time we have got *three* types of treatment. Therefore, the independent variable has three experimental *conditions or levels* — exercise, heat treatment and conventional therapy. Our design would look something like this:

Experimental Condition 1

| Pre-test measure of DV (physical condition) | New exercise regime (IV) | Post-test measure of DV (physical condition) |

Experimental Condition 2

| Pre-test measure of DV (physical condition) | Heat treatment (IV) | Post-test measure of DV (physical condition) |

Experimental Condition 3

| Pre-test measure of DV (physical condition) | Conventional therapy (IV) | Post-test measure of DV (physical condition) |

You could extend this further and add a control condition thus:

Experimental Condition 1
Experimental Condition 2
Experimental Condition 3
Control Condition

Compared on the dependent variable to assess whether there are any differences between the conditions

Or you could go on adding experimental conditions involving different forms of treatment.

In all these cases we still have only *one* independent variable, i.e. type of treatment, but we have varying numbers of experimental conditions or levels of it.

So, it should be clear by now that hypotheses which predict a relationship between one independent variable and a dependent variable may be tested by comparing:

a. one experimental condition and one control condition
b. two experimental conditions
c. two experimental conditions and one control condition
d. three experimental conditions
e. three experimental conditions and one control condition.
f. more than three experimental conditions etc.

Each of these designs requires a different statistical test to analyse the results, since unfortunately, there is no multi-purpose test for all experiments. Matching the design with the appropriate statistical test is something that we shall look at in Chapter 6.

CORRELATIONAL DESIGNS

Not all research has to take the form of manipulating an independent variable to see what effect it has on the dependent variable. Sometimes a researcher is not interested in looking for *differences* between groups or conditions in this way, but instead is concerned to find out whether two variables are *associated* or *related* (look back to pp. 39–40 to refresh your memory on the distinctions between experimental and correlational designs). Let's suppose we are interested in finding out whether there is a relationship between students' grades on clinical assessments and performance in theory exams since we have noticed that students who get high grades on one tend to get high grades on the other. Our hypothesis might be that 'There is a relationship between performance on clinical assessments and performance in theory exams, high marks on one being associated with high marks on the other.' The two variables are clinical assessment and theory exam performance.

However, one of the major differences in the research design needed to test this hypothesis is that the experimenter does **not** manipulate one of the variables, but simply takes a whole range of measures on one of the variables and assesses whether they are related to measures on the other variable. In our example, then, we might take a group of physiotherapy students and collect their clinical assessments and their theory exam marks to see if the two sets of scores are linked, e.g. high marks on one variable being associated with high marks on the other. Because the experimenter does not manipulate one variable, the concepts of Independent and Dependent Variable are not appropriate in correlational designs. Furthermore, because there is no manipulation of one variable and hence no measurement of the effect this has on the other variable, we cannot say in a correlational design which variable is cause and which effect. So returning to our example, we don't know whether clinical performance affects theory exam performance or vice versa. For instance, it may be that students who are good at clinical practice use their experience to answer their theory paper. Or it is possible that students who do well in theory use their knowledge in the clinical context. Alternatively, clinical performance and theory exam performance may both be related to a third variable. For example, good marks on both may be due to an 'easy' marker. Therefore, from any results we got from this study we do not actually know if:

practice affects theory

or

theory affects practice

or

another variable affects both theory and practice

You can see from this that because we cannot ascertain which variable is having an effect on the other, there cannot be an Independent or Dependent Variable. Even in correlational studies where we feel we could make an educated guess as to which variable is cause and which effect, we still cannot be *absolutely* sure. So, suppose we had some data which suggested there was a strong link between mental subnormality and epilepsy, such that the greater the degree of retardation, the greater the frequency of fits. We cannot necessarily conclude that epilepsy is the result of mental subnormality, since it is conceivable that the reverse may be true, such that the more fits someone has, the more damage is done to the brain. Alternatively, both epilepsy and mental subnormality may be the result of a third variable. So it is possible that:

mental subnormality leads to epilepsy

or

epilepsy leads to mental subnormality

or

mental subnormality and epilepsy are the result of a third variable, e.g. a brain tumour.

Because of the inability to state categorically which variable is cause and which is effect in a correlational design, many researchers prefer the certainty of experimental designs. However, because the experimenter is not involved in manipulating anything (such as types of treatment), the correlational design is often thought to be more acceptable ethically.

> **Key concepts**
>
> - Experimental designs have two variables in the hypothesis —
>   one Independent and one Dependent. The Independent
>   Variable is manipulated by the experimenter and the difference
>   this makes to the Dependent Variable is measured. Thus in
>   experimental designs we can ascertain cause and effect.
> - Correlational designs also have two variables in the hypothesis
>   but neither is manipulated. Therefore, there is no Independent
>   and no Dependent Variable. As a result it cannot be ascertained
>   which variable is having an effect on the other. All that can be
>   established is whether or not the scores on the two variables are
>   linked in some way.

It should be noted at this point that the degree to which each variable is
associated is determined using a statistical test appropriate for correlational
designs. We will deal with these in more detail in Chapter 11. Let's return
to our hypothesis and imagine that we have collected the clinical and theory
exam marks; the next step is to find out whether there is a significant
relationship between them. In order to do this, we use the appropriate
statistical test (see Ch. 11). When we have finished the calculations involved
in this test, we will end up with a number somewhere on a range from -1.0
through 0 to $+1.0$.

This figure is known as a *correlation coefficient*. The size of the correlation coefficient indicates the closeness of the relationship between the
two variables. The closer the figure is to -1 or $+1$, the closer the relationship, while the closer it is to 0 the weaker the relationship. This concept is
illustrated by the continuum below:

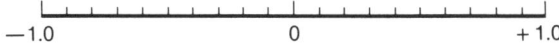

−1.0	0	+ 1.0

Fig. 19

Let's explore this idea a bit futher, using the hypothesis about the link between clinical assessments and theory exam marks. Supposing you had collected the clinical assessments and theory exam marks from 30 students (so you would have two scores for each student) you could plot their scores on a graph, known as a *scattergram*, to see if there is any association between the marks. You might end up with a scattergram which looks like this:

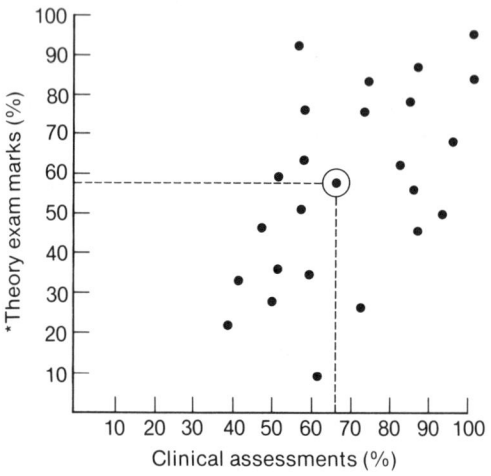

Fig. 20

In order to construct a scattergram, you would need to take each student's pair of scores (say, for the dot ringed above, 58% on the theory exam and 66% on the clinical assessment) and move along each relevant axis until you had located their score. You would make a mark at the intersection point.

Activity 11 (Answers on page 276)

To practise doing this, plot the following scores as a scattergram:
Hypothesis. There is a relationship between the number of cigarettes smoked daily and the rate of recovery following cardiothoracic surgery.

---

* In plotting a correlational graph, it does not matter which variable is plotted against the vertical axis and which against the horizontal one. However, should you ever wish to plot the data from an experimental design it is a convention that the Independent Variable scores are plotted along the horizontal axis and those from the Dependent Variable along the vertical axis.

Subject	No.. cigarettes	No. of days postop. to discharge
1	20	15
2	15	12
3	17	12
4	0	7
5	5	7
6	0	8
7	10	9
8	7	8
9	40	17
10	0	7

When you have plotted a scattergram you can see whether there *appears* to be a relationship between the two variables by the nature of the pattern of dots. If the dots show a general upward or downward slope, it is likely that there *is* a relationship between the two variables. So in the example about theory and practice marks, it seems that there *is* a relationship, because the *pattern of dots shows a general upward slope*. This is known as a *positive correlation*.

A positive correlation means that *high* scores on one variable are associated with *high* scores on the other and hence *low* scores on one variable and linked with *low* scores on the other. For example, there is a positive correlation between weight and hypertension, such that the *higher* the weight the *higher* the hypertension. So a scattergram pattern which shows a general upward slope like this:

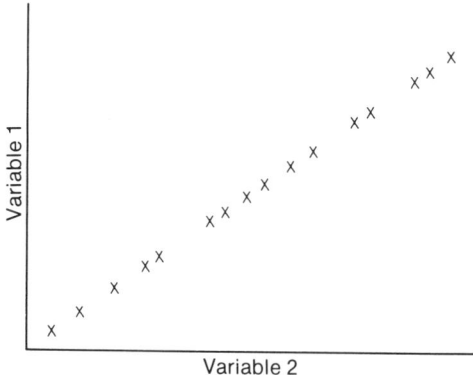

Variable 2

Fig. 21

indicates a positive correlation. It should be noted that the perfectly smooth upward slope on the above graph shows a perfect positive correlation (i.e. there is a one-to-one relationship between high scores on one variable and high scores on the other). However, perfect correlations are extremely rare, if they exist at all. But, the smoother and straighter the upward slope, the stronger the positive correlation between the two variable. A *positive* correlation would be represented on our continuum somewhere around the + 1.0 end:

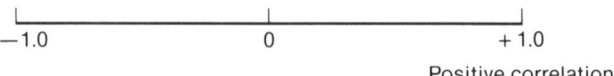

−1.0	0	+ 1.0

Positive correlation

Fig. 22

This figure would have been derived from a statistical analysis and the nearer to + 1, the stronger the relationship. This, however, is not the only sort of correlation that can occur. Sometimes it is possible that high scores on one variable are associated with low scores on the other. For example we might hypothesise a relationship between body weight of an arthritic patient and distance that can be walked, such that the *greater* the body weight the *shorter* the distance. Our data may look like this:

Patient	Weight (kg)	Distance (m)
1	74	12
2	59	20
3	64	15
4	67	15
5	72	10
6	80	5

Plotting these results on a scattergram, we end up with the following picture:

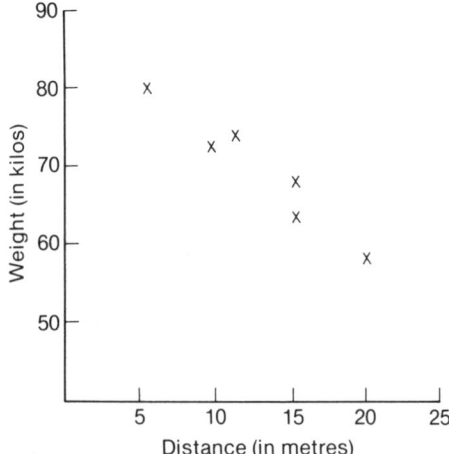

Fig. 23

There is a general *downward* slope in the pattern of dots. When this sort of pattern emerges, it suggests that *high* scores on one variable are associated with *low* scores on the other. This is known as a *negative correlation* and would be represented on our correlation coefficient near the − 1 end; the closer to − 1, the stronger the negative correlation.

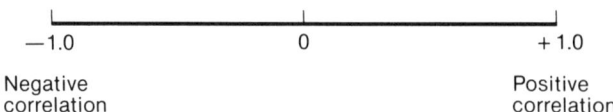

| −1.0 | 0 | + 1.0 |
| Negative correlation | | Positive correlation |

Fig. 24

On a scattergram, a negative correlation is indicated by the following pattern:

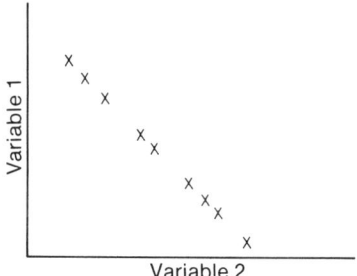

Fig. 25

(Again this shows a perfect negative correlation, which is very unlikely ever to occur.)

It is very important to note that a negative correlation does **not** mean **no** correlation. This is a point that confuses some students. A negative correlation indicates a relationship between high scores on one variable and low scores on the other, while no correlation means that there is no relationship at all between the two variables.

The following data demonstrate this:

Hypothesis   There is a relationship between the age of driver and the number of road traffic accidents.

Subject	Age	No. of road traffic accidents
1	19	1
2	30	2
3	57	0
4	41	5
5	25	4
6	32	1

Plotting these on a scattergram we get the following picture:

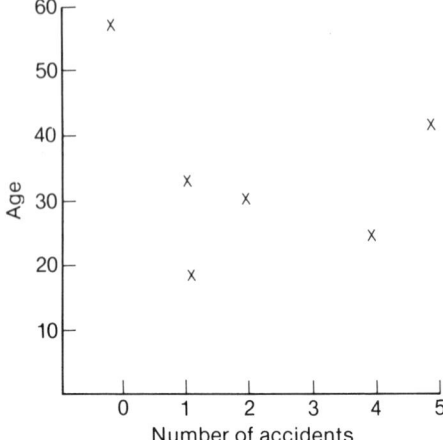

Fig. 26

This shows a fairly random scattering of dots, suggesting there is no link between the variables of age and the number of road traffic accidents.

In this case the correlation coefficient score from our statistical analysis would be around 0:

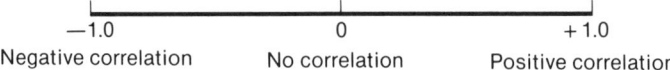

Fig. 27

Key concepts

- Positive correlations indicate that high scores on one variable are associated with high scores on the other
    - they are represented by an upward slope on a scattergram
    - they have a correlation coefficient near + 1, with the closer the coefficient to + 1, the stronger the positive correlation.
- Negative correlations indicate that high scores on one variable are associated with low scores on the other
    - they are represented by a downward slope on a scattergram
    - they have a correlation coefficient of around − 1, with the nearer the coefficient to − 1, the stronger the negative correlation.
- No correlation indicates that there is no relationship between the scores on the two variables
    - they are represented by random clusterings on a scattergram with no obvious direction to the pattern
    - they have a correlation coefficient of around 0, with the closer the coefficient to 0, the weaker the relationship between the two variables.

Activity 12 (Answers on page 277)

1. Look at the following hypotheses and state whether they suggest positive or negative correlations between the variables. Also state how they would be represented on a scattergram and where on a scale of -1 to $+1$ the correlation coefficient would be.

  (i) The older the patient, the longer the recovery time following lower leg amputation.
 (ii) The further from an outpatients' physiotherapy department a patient lives, the less the likelihood of keeping an appointment.
(iii) The lower the 'A'-level results of physiotherapy students, the lower the mock exam mark in the final year.
(iv) The higher the intake of dietary fibre, the lower the incidence of diverticulitis.

2. Look at the following correlation coefficients and rank them from the *strongest* relationship to the *weakest*:

$$-0.73 \quad -0.42 \quad +0.61 \quad +0.21 \quad -0.17 \quad +0.09$$

It should also be noted that if you do find that the two variables are correlated together, you are able to make predictions about one variable from information about the other. Therefore, if you found that two variables were negatively correlated, you could predict high scores on one variable from knowledge of low scores on the other and vice versa. Equally, if you found that two variables were positively correlated, you could predict high scores on one variable from a knowledge of high scores on the other or low scores could be predicted for one variable from a knowledge of low scores on the other.

We have already said that the nature of the scattergram and the correlation coefficient indicate the strength of the relationship between the two variables and that there is no such thing as a perfect correlation. Therefore how smooth must the scattergram slope be and how close must the correlation coefficient be to $+$ or -1 before we decide that there is a relationship? Will $+0.63$ do? or -0.54? Because we cannot make an arbitrary decision like this, after we have calculated the correlation coefficient using a statistical test, we use a set of statistical tables to see whether the correlation coefficient is sufficiently big to indicate that the relationship between the two variables is significant. This will also depend on how many subjects you have used in your project. We will deal with these concepts in more detail in Chapter 11.

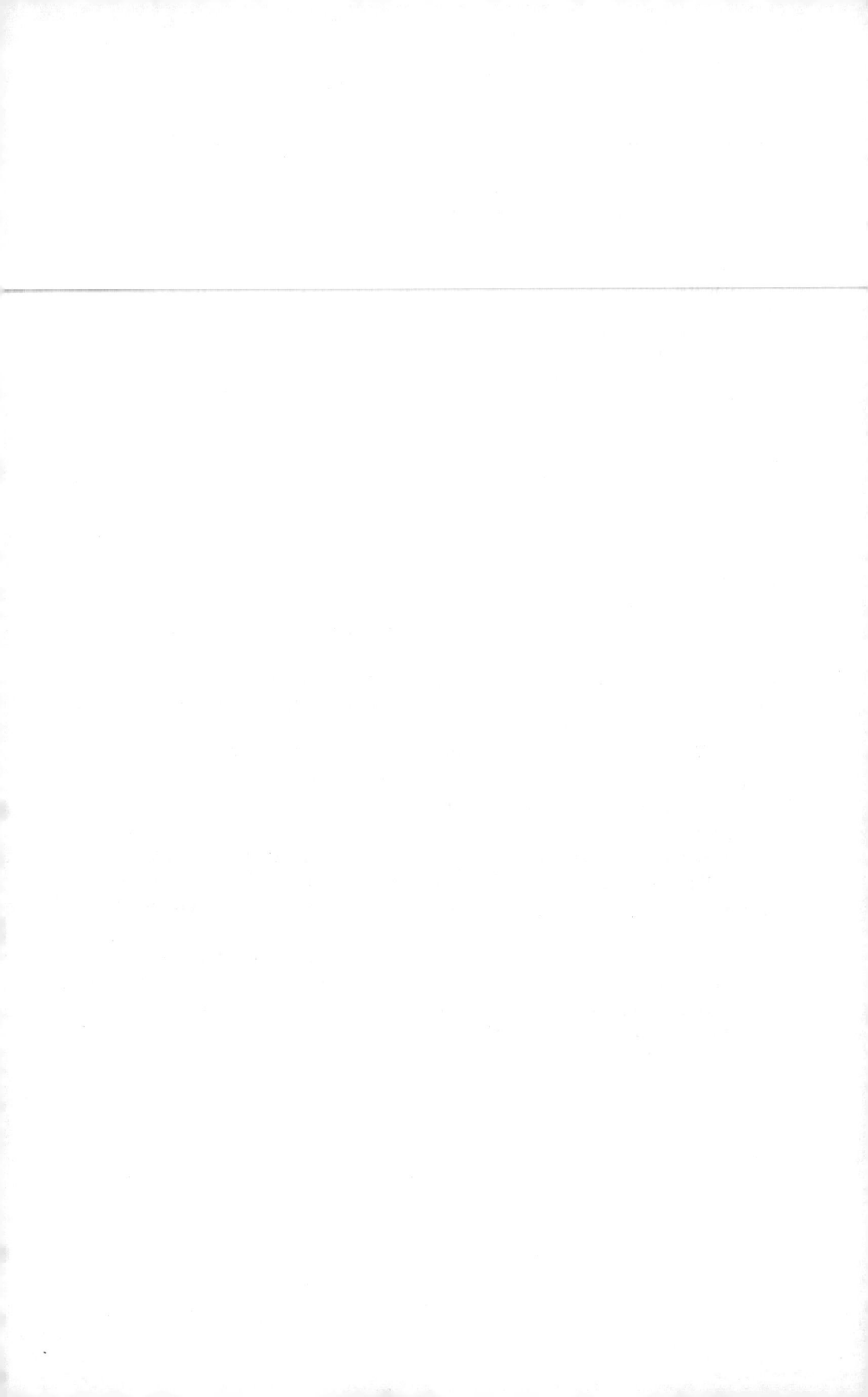

4

Further aspects of research design

When you carry out any research you will almost certainly recruit people (perhaps patients or colleagues) to take part in it. These people who take part in experiments are called *subjects* — sometimes referred to as *Ss*. You will always have to decide what sort of subjects you need in your research, for instance, trainee physiotherapists, cystic fibrosis patients, elderly amputees. But whoever you decide to use, there is a very important point to note — you don't want your results to apply *only* to the small group or *sample* of people you used in your experiment as you need to be able to *generalise* your results. This is a crucial feature of research and central to the topic of inferential statistics. For example, supposing you had compared the lung capacity of 20 cystic fibrosis patients treated by clapping with 20 treated by breathing exercises and had found better results with the exercises group. It is important that these results do not *just* apply to the 20 subjects you used in your experiment, but that they are very likely to apply to other cystic fibrosis patients. The point here is that if your results can be generalised in this way, then *predictions* can be made — and this is another essential feature of research. So, when confronted by a new cystic fibrosis patient you can *predict* that breathing exercises are more likely to be effective than clapping on the basis of the generalisability of the results from your research.

But, short of carrying out your experiment on huge numbers of cystic fibrosis patients, how can you ascertain that your results *are* generalisable? We have already touched on this issue when the topic of inferential statistics was introduced; if you recall, inferential statistics allow the researcher to use a small sample of people in an experiment, and from the results of these experiments to *infer* that the same findings would apply to the larger population from which the sample comes. Now in order to be able to make this assumption, you must ensure that the sample you selected for study is:

a. sufficiently large to ensure that it reflects the larger group or population from which it is derived. Let's consider the situation whereby the district physiotherapist is thinking about altering the number of hours in the day shift. If she asks *one* physiotherapist out of the 30 under her, then it is less likely that she will receive a view which reflects the opinion of the whole group (or *population*) than if she asks 15 of the 30. In other words the number of subjects you select for study must be sufficiently big for you to be able to generalise the results from your experiment. What does this mean in practice? Well, although opinions on this vary, it is usually considered that 12 subjects per group or condition is the minimum number required. Of course, if you're dealing with von Recklinghausen's syndrome it will be unlikely that you will get as many as 12. But aim for a minimum of 12 subjects per group or condition. There are, however, situations where more subjects are required. Where this is the case, it will be pointed out in the relevant chapter. Similarly, in some of the illustrations quoted in later chapters, fewer than 12 subjects are used. This has been done simply for ease of calculation.

b. representative of the population from which they come and so are *typical*.

The easiest way to ensure typicality is to select your subjects *randomly*, for instance putting the names of *all* the cystic fibrosis patients you might have access to in a hat and randomly selecting 20, or tossing a coin. This point will be referred to again later in the chapter. Before moving on though, it is important to recognise that you cannot always select your subjects randomly because there are insufficient numbers of particular patient types. If this is the case, then you must be aware of the limitations on generalising the results from such a study.

Nonetheless, whatever sort of subjects are involved in your study, you will need to decide how to use them in the research design and this decision is a crucial one when designing a piece of research.

For example, if you look back to the hypothesis given on page 43 where it was predicted that physiotherapists who attended a psychology course developed more tolerant attitudes than those who did not attend, you will see that to test this hypothesis it was suggested that two groups of physiotherapists were selected, one of which attended the course, and the other of which did not. In other words, two *different* groups of physiotherapists were used, one in the control condition and one in the experimental condition. However, not all hypotheses are best tested by comparing different groups of subjects in this way; sometimes it is more appropriate to use just *one* group of subjects and to measure them on two or more occasions.

When two or more different groups of subjects are used and compared in a project, it is called an *unrelated, between* or *different subject* design. When just one group of subjects is used in all conditions it is called a *related, within* or *same subject design*. We will look at each of these more closely.

1. DIFFERENT SUBJECT DESIGNS (ALSO KNOWN AS UNRELATED SUBJECT OR BETWEEN SUBJECT DESIGNS)

It was said earlier that hypotheses could often be tested in different ways, using different experimental designs, and that it was the job of the experimenter to decide on the most suitable design for a particular hypothesis. However, for some hypotheses there is really only one obvious way to test them. If you look again at the hypothesis about physiotherapists' attendance on a psychology course, two different groups of physiotherapists were used, one as a control condition and one as an experimental condition.

The design looked like this:

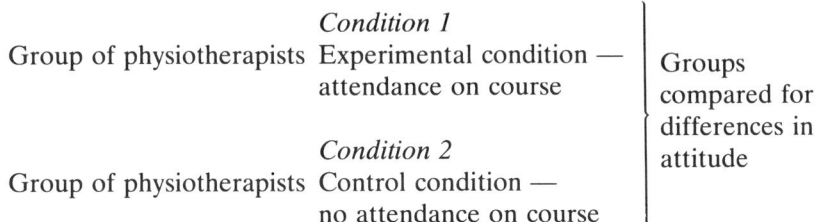

At the end of the experiment the attitude change of the two groups would be compared to see if, in fact, the group who had attended the course became more tolerant.

This is a typical example of the sort of hypothesis which requires a different-subject design since it would have been totally inappropriate to use just one group for both conditions. If we think about this idea a bit more closely, it becomes clear that if we *had* selected just one group of physiotherapists, to be both the control (no course) condition and the experimental (attendance on course) condition, all sorts of problems emerge. Let's explore this a bit further. There are two possible ways of carrying out this experiment, using just one group of subjects.
You could either send your group of physiotherapists

a. on a course for 3 months (experimental condition)
           followed by
  'no course' for 3 months (control condition)
                 or
b. on 'no course' for 3 months (control condition)
           followed by
  a course for 3 months (experimental condition)

You can see from this that although there are control and experimental conditions in each design, the results for each would be contaminated because the group had done both conditions. For example, in the first design, if we did find that there was a significant attitude change after going on a course for 3 months and that there was no further change after the 'no course' condition what could we *really* conclude about the control condition? It may be that the control condition had no effect because the group's attitudes had changed as far as they could by the end of the course or because the control condition was a time for *consolidating* the attitude change already experienced. Alternatively, if we found that there *was* a change during the control condition this may be due to the continued effect of the course, or the effects of 3 months more time and experience — but we wouldn't know *which*.

In the second design, any change in attitude found after doing the course might simply be due to the combined effects of the control and experimental conditions or the passage of time on the experience, opinions and attitudes of these subjects and not to the course. In other words, whatever the *order* these designs adopt, any results obtained would have more than one explanation because we have contaminated the outcome by subjecting the subjects to both conditions. This is known as an *order* effect and will be discussed in more detail later in the chapter. Therefore, a hypothesis like this one requires a different subject design in order to eliminate the confounding effects of participating in both conditions.

There are many other hypotheses in physiotherapy research which necessitate using two or more different groups of subjects. For example, any comparisons of different races, ages, sexes, type of patient etc. all mean that different subjects have to be used. For example, if you wanted to compare muscle tone of Asian and West Indian children, you would have to use one group of Asians and another group of West Indians. One subject group is quite obviously inappropriate here, since it is impossible for someone to be of both racial origins.

While it is sometimes essential to use different groups of subjects in your experiment, there is a major disadvantage in the design: that of individual differences among the subjects. If we look at the example regarding differences in muscle tone between Asian and West Indian children, it is quite possible that some children would not really understand what they have to do in the experiment, others may just have had flu' and so be feeling weaker anyway, others may be really motivated to please the experimenter, yet others may be frightened. All these factors may influence how a subject performs in an experiment and so will affect the results. For example, the child who is frightened of the experimenter and the situation may have increased muscle tone due to fear. Therefore, his performance score may be high for reasons other than inherent muscle tone. While these individual difference *may* be evenly distributed among all the groups thereby cancelling the effects out, it is also likely that more of the individual differences that affect the results may occur in *only* one of the groups and thus will artificially distort the results.

The problem of individual differences can be partly overcome by ensuring that the subjects are *randomised*. Randomisation can mean one of two things. Firstly, it can mean selecting a group of subjects (e.g. hip replacement patients) and randomly allocating half of them to one treatment and half to the other, in order to compare the effects. Obviously, this cannot be done in our example about muscle tone, since it would not be possible to select a group of children and randomly allocate them to being Asian or West Indian. Here randomness means something different — that the subjects in each group should be a random, and therefore typical, selection of the group they represent. In other words, the children in the Asian group should be typical of Asian children as a whole, and not all *particularly* weak, strong, fit, athletic, motivated, awkward or anything else. The same should be true of the children in West Indian group. The ways in which random selection can be achieved is outlined in Chapter 2 and also throughout this chapter.

Key concepts

When two or more different groups of subjects are used in an experiment it is called

> an unrelated subject design
> or
> a between subject design
> or
> a different subject design.

The *advantages* of this design is that it can overcome any problems associated with the order of conditions and it is also essential when 'fixed' differences such as races, sex, ages, types of patient are being compared. However, its major *disadvantage* is that individual differences among the subjects may distort the results. This can be partially overcome by randomising the selection of subjects and their allocation to conditions.

---

2. SAME SUBJECT DESIGNS (ALSO KNOWN AS RELATED–SUBJECT OR WITHIN–SUBJECT DESIGNS)

Some hypotheses, however, are not suited to using designs with different subjects in each condition. Some hypotheses are more suited to being tested by designs which use only *one* group of subjects, but this group is measured under *all* the conditions and its performance in each condition is compared.

For example, you might be interested in looking at the level of confidence a group of elderly patients had in uniformed vs non-uniformed physiotherapists. Here you would randomly select a group of patients and ask them to indicate how confident they felt (a) when being treated by a uniformed physiotherapist and (b) when being treated by a non-uniformed physiotherapist. The design would look like this:

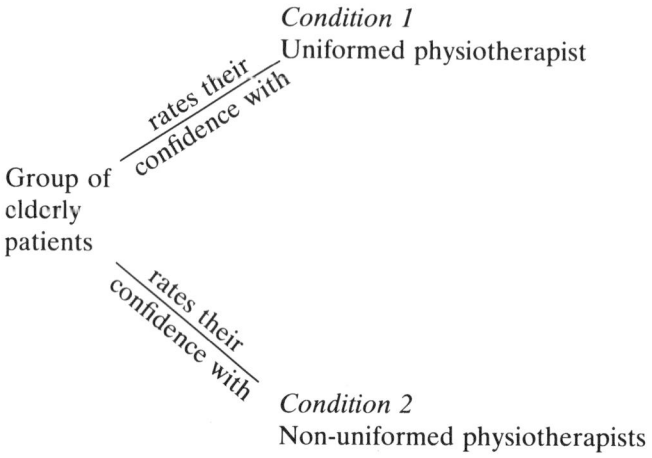

Thus, *one* group of subjects is tested under all conditions and the two sets of ratings are compared to see if there is any difference between them. It would be inappropriate here to use two groups of patients, one to rate the uniformed physiotherapists and the other to rate the non-uniformed, because the groups may differ inherently in a number of ways which would affect the outcome of the results. For example, one group may be generally more confident anyway, may love all uniforms, or may try harder to please the experimenter by inflating their ratings etc. Hence, there may be basic individual differences between the two groups which might affect the results. However, if we use just one group of patients then whatever their idio-syncrasies and personal characteristics, they will at least be constant over both ratings. Therefore, one important advantage of a same subject design is the fact that it overcomes the problem of individual differences inherent in different subject designs. Because of this, it is especially useful in 'before and after' type experiments, where the researcher wants to look at the effects of a treatment procedure on a group of subjects.

However, it too has its snags. If we look at the last example, supposing we gave *all* the subjects the uniformed-rating task first, and the non-uniformed rating task second, it is quite conceivable that on the first task they didn't quite understand what was required of them and so filled in the questionaire using the wrong criteria, while by the second task they had realised what they had to do. This may well distort the results. Alternatively, it could be argued that by the time the second task had to be completed, the subjects were bored or tired and so filled in lower confidence ratings. In other words, the results may have been affected by the *order* in which the tasks were carried out. Therefore to overcome this, half the subject should do Task A first, followed by Task B, while for the remaining subjects, the order would be reversed. This is called *counterbalancing* and is discussed more fully later in the chapter.

> **Key concept**
>
> When one group of subjects is tested or measured on all the conditions and their performance compared it is known as a
>
> related subject design
> or
> same subject design
> or
> within subject design.
>
> The *advantage* of this design is that it eliminates the distorting effects of individual subject differences. However, it has two *disadvantages*: firstly, it cannot be used when 'fixed' differences such as sex, race, type of ailment are being compared and secondly, any effects deriving from the *order* of the conditions may have to be counterbalanced.

3. MATCHED SUBJECT DESIGNS

One way of overcoming all the disadvantages of both different and same subject designs is to use *two* groups of subjects who are matched on a number of characteristics. Let's take an example. Suppose you wanted to compare the recovery times of leg fractures resulting from RTAs and leg fractures resulting from sports injuries. Obviously you cannot use a same subject design, since a patient's fracture cannot simultaneously be due to an RTA and sports injury, and if you use a different subject design, you might find a number of individual differences in the subjects which predisposed one group to recover more quickly than the other. For example, the sports injuries patients may be younger, male, fitter and stronger, whereas the RTA patients may be less fit, older, diabetic and include females. All these factors may be influence recovery rates. In such cases, then, it is necessary to try to identify the personal characteristics of the subjects which may bias the outcome of the experiment and to ensure that the groups are matched on these factors.

The way in which the matching is carried out involves firstly, identifying all the possible individual characteristics which may influence the results and then to select a subject (for example, an RTA patient) and assess how he rates on these characteristics. For example, in this case, you might note his age, sex, degree of fitness (perhaps by heart rate, pulse rate, blood pressure), previous fractures to the leg (and anything else you feel may bias the results). You must then find another patient in the sports injuries category who is the same age, sex, has the same fitness ratings, has had the same number of previous fractures to the leg and has other characteristics similar to the RTA patient. Therefore, in terms of the personal characteristics which are likely to influence the results from the experiment, each pair of subjects is like identical twins, with the only difference between them being the way in which the fracture occurred. Thus, for every subject in one group, there is an 'identical twin' in the other.

When you are involved in comparing 'non-fixed' groups, e.g. the effects of the different treatments, you can match up a pair of subjects first and then randomly allocate one subject to one treatment and the 'twin' to the other treatment. Because of the similarity of the subjects, matched designs are treated like same subject designs for the purposes of statistical analysis. Similarly, as with same subject designs, the matched design overcomes the problem of individual differences, because of the 'twinning' of the subjects. Yet the matched design has all the advantages of a different subject design, since 'fixed' groups can be compared and there need be no order effects.

So why don't we always use matched designs if they're so good? I'm sure you will have realised already that it is often extremely difficult to match pairs of subjects in this way, usually because there are limited numbers of suitable subjects to choose from. Even if we allow ourselves a little leeway, say by matching an RTA patient aged 30 with a sports injury patient aged 28, there may still be many important differences between the subject pair that we either cannot identify or cannot match for, e.g. biochemical composition of bones and blood that affect healing rates. Thus, while these designs are theoretically very desirable, in practical terms they are extremely difficult to implement properly. It must be stressed that it is *not* adequate simply to select 20 RTAs and 20 sports injury patients, all of whom are male and under 40 and say that you've matched them. For every subject in one group, there must be a 'twinned' subject in the other, matched on all the relevant variables which may influence the outcome of the experiment. Therefore, because of the difficulties involved in matching people, caused largely through our lack of knowledge of which factors are relevant, it is usually desirable to use a same-subject design in preference to a matched subject design. As one statistician says:

> A matching design is only as good as the Experimenter's ability to determine how to match the pairs, and this ability is frequently very limited.
>
> Sidney Siegel (1956)

Key concept

Matched designs involve selecting pairs of subjects, matched on any variable which may influence the outcome of the experiment, and allocating one of the pair to one condition and one to the other. This design has all the advantages of same and different subject designs, but has the major disadvantage that it is very difficult to match subjects in this way because firstly it is not always possible to find subjects who are sufficiently similar, and secondly, you can never be sure that you have matched pairs of subjects on all the factors that may influence the results.

SOURCES OF ERROR IN RESEARCH

There are a number of potential sources of bias or *error* in an experiment which may distort your results and which need to be controlled for. We will look at each of these separately.

Order effects

When a piece of research is carried out which follows an *experimental* design the experimenter manipulates the independent variable and measures the effect of this on the dependent variable, in the hope that altering the IV will have a significant effect on the DV. Changes in the DV are called the *experimental effect*. Let's take an example. Suppose you had hypothesised that students perform worse on a neurological placement than on an orthopaedic placement during their second year of training, in other words you are predicting a relationship between type of placement (IV) and performance (DV). To test this, you set up the following experiment:

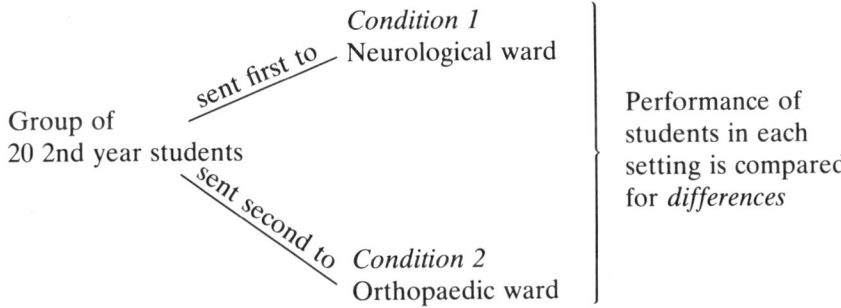

The performances in both placements are compared (using the appropriate statistical test) to see if one differs significantly from the other. Let us assume that you did in fact find that students seem to do better on orthopaedic placements — can we conclude that the results are the effect of some inherent difficulty associated with neurological physiotherapy? Or might there be some other explanations?

One obvious alternative explanation that we've already touched on and you've probably thought of, relates to the sequence of the placements. If the students' *first* placement is on a neurological ward and their subsequent placement is on an orthopaedic ward, it is conceivable that their improved performance in the latter case may be due simply to the fact that it *was* second. In other words, the students may do better on *any* second placement (regardless of its nature) because they are more confident, more skilled, more familiar with hospital routines etc. — they are more *practised*. Hence, this is known as a *practice effect*. It is, of course, equally likely that students do *worse* on their second placement because they are more jaundiced, more tired, less motivated etc. This is known as a *fatigue effect*.

Regardless of which argument you support, the general issue is the same — that *order effects*, rather than the nature of the placement itself, could be affecting students' performance. Order effects are a common problem in experiments where *one* group of subjects is compared on two or more conditions. In order to get round this problem, a technique called *counterbalancing* is used, where *half* the subjects do activity A first, followed by activity B, while the other half do activity B first, followed by activity A. In our example, then, 10 students would do their neurological placement first, followed by the orthopaedic placement, while for the remaining 10 the order would be reversed. At the end of the study, *all* the neurological ratings would be compared with *all* the orthopaedic ratings. You can select which students do which placement first by a number of methods — the first 10 students alphabetically, the first 10 names pulled out of a hat, alternate names alphabetically. While it doesn't really matter which method you use, do try to ensure that the students are *randomly* allocated. Don't put all your worst students into neurology first just to prove your point!

So, by counterbalancing in this way, any bias in the results due to order effects is balanced out. One point is important here: we cannot eliminate order effects totally, because one activity *must* precede the other in designs like this. All we can do is to balance out the order effects *as far as possible.*

Key concepts

If one group of subjects has to be measured in all the conditions then the order in which they do these conditions may influence the results. For example, they may perform *better* on the last activity because of *practice effects*, or they may perform *worse* on the last activity because of *fatigue effects*. In order to eliminate these sources of bias, the order in which the subjects carry out the activities should be *counterbalanced*, such that half the subjects does activity A first, followed by B, while for the remainder, the order is reversed.

So, one possible explanation for the results from this experiment (and any other which involves a same subject design) lies in the possibility of order effects. However, even if you had counterbalanced these, there are still other variables which could account for your results.

Experimenter bias effects

Suppose — like all experimenters — you are very committed to your research and are very keen that your hypothesis will be supported, in this case, that students *will* do worse on neurological wards. It is conceivable that in your anxiety and enthusiasm to obtain the predicted outcome, you will unwittingly influence the results. I don't mean by this that you will cook the books, but that *unawares*, you may use a slightly different set of criteria when assessing the students on each placement perhaps ignoring some negative things on the orthopaedic placement, or putting more emphasis on others while carrying out the evaluation. In other words, you may have a set of expectations about the outcome of the experiment which will influence what you perceive, how you behave etc. Such influences are very common and are known as *experimenter bias* effects. Other types of experimenter bias include the *personal* characteristics of the experimenter, such as status, sex, class, race, age and so on, all of which may have some effect on the subjects and their performance.

It should be emphasised that normally such experimenter influences are quite unintentional and unconscious, but there is a great deal of documented evidence to show that they exist. How can we get round this problem? The usual solution is to operate a *double-blind* procedure, whereby you ask someone who does not know what your hypothesis is to collect your data — in this case, to assess the students. Because they are not aware of what you have predicted, they will also not know how the students are meant to behave in each placement and so their evaluation of the students' performance should be much more objective. This sort of double-blind procedure is very common in medical research, particularly when carrying out drug trials. In these cases, one group of patients is given the drug, while another group is given a placebo. But neither the doctors assessing the outcome nor the patients themselves know who has been given which. In this way, the results cannot be biased by expectations.

Key concepts

Sometimes experimenters unwittingly influence the outcome of their experiment by the way in which they behave, appear or interact with the subjects. This is known as *experimenter bias*. To overcome this sort of problem in your research, you should use a *double-blind* procedure, whereby you ask someone who is absolutely unaware of what your hypothesis is to collect your data. In this way, any bias due to expectations and predictions will be eliminated.

However, there are still other variables which may influence our results, besides the manipulation of the IV even if we control for order and experimenter bias effects. These are called *constant errors* and *random errors*. Let's look at constant errors first.

Constant errors

Constant errors are all the possible sources of bias and influence that will affect the results in a constant and predictable way. If we go back to our example of comparing students' performance in two placements, we can identify a number of potential sources of constant error. Suppose the neurological ward had 50 patients, 2 qualified physiotherapists and 10 students, while the orthopaedic ward had 25 patients, 5 qualified staff and 10 students. Under such conditions, it is quite possible that students do less well on the neurological ward because (a) of greater patient to staff ratios, which would increase workload, pressure, tension etc. and (b) they have fewer qualified physiotherapists available to teach and support them. Therefore, their poor performance may be the direct result of these variables and not to do with problems inherent to neurological work. Also, the superintendent physiotherapist at the neurological hospital may dislike the disruption caused by students and so may provide less constructive tuition and guidance. The neurological placement may also involve a more arduous journey (students arrive feeling fatigued), or longer shifts or any one of a number of other problems. Note that each of these factors can be called a *constant* error because of the predictable way in which they would distort the results. For example, high patient/staff ratios are more likely to depress students' performance than improve it and so the effect of this variable is *constant*; less tuition will also depress, not improve, performance, as will fatigue. Thus, each of these factors will have a similar effect on all the students and so will distort the results in a constant, predictable way.

It is your job as a researcher to try to identify all the possible sources of constant error in your experiment and either to eliminate or control them. If you leave any constant error uncontrolled then your results may be explained by that, rather than by the manipulation of the IV. Taking the constant errors quoted as examples here, we can eliminate or control them in the following way:

Constant error	Solution
1. Different patient/staff ratios	Ensure both placements have comparable ratios
2. Different numbers of qualified staff to act as tutors	Ensure student/qualified staff are the same in each placement
3. Different attitudes of superintendents resulting in restricted supervision times	Ensure students in each placement receive same amounts of clinical instruction
4. Different journey lengths	Either select placements which are equidistant or arrange transport to neuro hospital such that travelling times and problems are similar
5. Different shift times/lengths	Ensure students in each placement work the same number of hours at similar times of day

In other words, you must *standardise* all aspects of the experimental situation in each placement.

Thus, when designing an experiment you must try to highlight all the factors which will bias your results in a similar, constant way and then make attempts to eliminate or control them by standardising the situation and procedures in each condition.

Random errors

Random errors are not as easy to deal with. As their name suggests, they are random — randomly occurring, randomly distributed and with a random and unpredictable impact on the results. If we look back to our example, we identified some factors that would influence our results in a very predictable way, but there are other factors — the random errors — which will obscure our results in a totally variable or *chance* way.

For example, the moods of the patients, staff and students will all have an effect on performance. If *all* the neurological patients were *always* in a bad mood and *all* the orthopaedic patients *always* in a good mood their moods would influence the results in a predictable way and so would be classified as constant errors. But moods aren't like that — they fluctuate up and down and interact with other people's behaviour, mood and attitudes. As a result they cannot be eliminated or controlled. Transitory changes in health among the patients, staff and students, personalities, attitudes, variation in motivation are all examples of random error — factors which will obscure the results in an unpredictable, chance way and about which we can do very little.

The only real precaution that we can take against random errors is to ensure *as far as possible* that the people involved in our research are drawn randomly from the population they represent. Therefore, our students should be fairly typical of physiotherapy students as a whole and not particularly deviant, disturbed, problematic, good, able or anything else. The neurological patients should be fairly typical of neurology patients as a whole and not particularly unusual, ill, well, independent, dependent, irascible, helpful etc., and similarly with the orthopaedic patients and staff. In this way the random errors should be fairly evenly distributed across both the placements, and therefore should (at least theoretically) affect the students' performance in each setting in a similar, if random, way.

One other point is important here — if your subjects can be *randomly allocated* to conditions (e.g., to different treatments, or in this case, allocating students to a particular *order* of placements) so much the better, because the random errors should then be evenly distributed. Randomisation can be achieved by tossing a coin, drawing names out of hat, taking every alternative patient/student/physio — there is no great mystique to it!

Key concepts

- *Constant errors* are those factors that distort the results in a constant or predictable way. They can be eliminated or controlled by *standardising* the procedures and conditions.
- *Random errors* are those factors which obscure the results in a random or unpredictable way. They cannot be eliminated, although random selection and allocation of subjects will distribute them evenly across conditions (at least theoretically).

Activity 13 (Answers on pages 277–278)

Look at the following hypotheses and identify the sources of constant and random error and their solutions:

H_1: Men are more likely to suffer respiratory complications following cardiothoracic surgery than are women.

Constant error	Solution	Random error	Solution

H_1: Outpatients' clinics achieve better recovery rates for leg fractures than specific sports injuries clinics.

Constant error	Solution	Random error	Solution

Probabilities

If we cannot get rid of random errors, how can we be sure that the results from our experiment are due to some real and significant relationship between the variables, as predicted in the hypothesis, and *not* to the obscuring effect of random errors? The answer to this lies in the use of statistical tests. When we use a statistical test to analyse a set of results, we end up with a numerical value. This value is looked up in a set of probability tables, to give us a probability or *p value*, which is expressed either as a *decimal* (e.g. 0.01) or as a *percentage* (e.g. 1%). *This p value tells us how probable it is that the results from our experiment are due to random errors.* It is very important to understand and remember this, as it is the basis of all statistical analyses.

Because this *p* value tells us how likely it is that the results from the experiment are due to random error (and *not* to the real and consistent relationship predicted in your hypothesis) then the *smaller* the *p* value, the *smaller* the possibility that random error or chance factors can account for your results. Therefore, by implication, the *smaller* the possibility that your results are due to random error, then the *greater* the possibility that they are due to the relationship you predicted in your hypothesis. Thus, the smaller the *p* value, the greater the inferred support or *significance* of your experimental hypothesis. Do bear in mind that it is *highly* unlikely that you will ever get 100% support for your hypothesis, and so *p* will always have a value greater than 0. If your *p* value is very low, then you can reject the null (no relationship) hypothesis, and conclude the experimental hypothesis has been supported. (Remember! When we carry out an experiment we do *not* set out to support our experimental hypothesis *directly*, but instead, we try to reject the null (no relationship) hypothesis — see Ch. 3).

Probability values, as was noted earlier, can be expressed either as a percentage or as a decimal. Therefore, if our *p* value was 5% (or 0.05) then we could say that there is a 5% chance that the results are due to random error (this is sometimes expressed as a 5% error margin or error rate) and by implication, that there is 95% support for your hypothesis.

Let's take another example. Suppose you had obtained a p value of 3% for your results. This means that there is a 3/100 chance that your results are due to the effects of chance or random error factors, and a 97/100 chance that are due to the effects of the real and consistent relationship you predicted in your hypothesis.

Activity 14 (Answers on page 278)

Look at the following p values and order them in terms of greatest inferred support for your experimental hypothesis. (Greatest support on the left, to least support on the right.)

$p = 5\%$ $p = 19\%$ $p = 7\%$ $p = 0.01\%$ $p = 15\%$ $p = 3\%$

When you have done this, convert each p value to a decimal.

> **Key concepts**
>
> When you carry out a statistical analysis, you end up with a numerical value which you look up in a set of probability tables to give you a p value. The p value tells you how likely it is that the results from your experiment are due to random error or chance. The *smaller* the p value, the *stronger* the support for your hypothesis. P values are expressed as percentages or decimals.

Activity 15 (Answers on page 278)

Suppose you saw the following p values in some medical article, what do they mean in terms of the possibility of chance or random factors being responsible for the results?

	% support for hypothesis	% probability that the results are due to chance
$p = 1\%$		
$p = 7\%$		
$p = 3\%$		
$p = 5\%$		
$p = 0.5\%$		

Significant levels

It was said earlier that if your p value was very small you could reject the null (no relationship) hypothesis and conclude that your experimental hypothesis has been supported by the results. When the null hypothesis is rejected in this way, the results are said to be *significant*. But how small must your p value be before you can conclude that your results are significant? There is no simple answer to this as it depends upon the nature of the experiment you've carried out.

For example, suppose you had hypothesised that a new form of treatment was much more effective for bronchitic patients' vital capacity than the standard breathing exercises. In order to carry out this research you randomly allocate 20 patients to the new treatment and 20 to the old treatment, and after a month you compare their vital capacities, using the appropriate statistical test. Let's assume your resulting p value is 5%, this means that there is an error rate of 5/100. Put another way, if you treated 100 bronchitis patients with the new treatment, 95 would improve as a result of the treatment but 5 would not (or if they did, it would be due to chance and not to the effects of the treatment). If nothing too awful happened to these 5 patients when they failed to respond to treatment, you would probably be quite happy to treat every bronchitis patient with the new treatment, since there is only a 5% error margin. However, supposing that the new treatment, when it *did not* work, proved fatal, and killed the 5 patients instead. With this outcome you would probably require a *much* smaller error margin in your results — perhaps 1 error in every 1000 or 10 000 — before you recommended the new treatment. In other words, the *effect* of the error determines how small your p value must be before you can conclude your results are significant. We could compare this to placing a bet on Grand National Day. Supposing you've looked at the horses, and you've decided to place a bet on a particular horse — you've unwittingly formulated an hypothesis that there is a relationship between this horse and final placing. If you're only going to put 10p on this horse, you won't mind a fairly large error margin (or p value) because losing 10p is not too disastrous. However, if you've placed all your life-savings and assets on this horse, then you want to be very sure that it's going to win. In other words, you will want to ensure a *small* error margin before you bet, since if you *are* wrong, the effects will be devastating.

The error margin or p value you decide upon in an experiment is called the *level of significance*. It is so-called because when you look up the results of your statistical analysis in a set of probability tables, you will find the p value for your results. If this p value is equal to or smaller than the significance level you have selected as being appropriate for your research, then your results are said to be *significant*. This means that you can reject the null (no relationship) hypothesis and accept that your experimental hypothesis has been supported. If the p value is *larger* than the significance level you have selected, your results are classed as *not significant*, which means you cannot reject the null hypothesis.

Therefore, it is up to you, the experimenter, to state what significance level you think is appropriate for a particular piece of research and the significance level you finally select will reflect the nature of your experiment. All this seems to leave the field wide open for you. However, a good rule-of-thumb if you're *not* doing anything that may have a disastrous outcome if you're wrong, is to use a cut-off point or significance level of *5%. So if you obtain a p value of 5% or less, then you can conclude that your results are significant and that your experimental hypothesis has been supported.*

This point will be referred to again later.

Key concepts

The p value states the probability of your results being due to chance or random error. If the p value is very small (that is, there is a very small margin of error in your results) you can conclude that your results are *significant*. This means you can reject the null (no difference) hypothesis and conclude that your experimental hypothesis has been supported. The experimenter decides upon how small the error margin must be before the results are said to be significant. The size of the error margin is called the *significance level*. The decision about the size of the significance level is based on the effects of the error. If the error is likely to be disastrous, then the significance level is reduced. If the effects are not likely to be terrible, then the significance level can be increased. A good rule-of-thumb is to use a 5% significance level as long as you are not doing anything dangerous.

5

Levels of measurement

Whatever sort of research you're interested in, you will be involved in *measuring* something, e.g. exam performance, distance walked, vital capacity, range of movement and so on. These measurements form your data or results. If we look at the above examples a bit more carefully, we can see that each of them involves a different sort of measurement:

— exam performance may be measured as marks out of 20 or 100
— distance walked may be measured in yards and feet
— vital capacity may be measured in ccs
— range of movement may be measured in degrees.

You can doubtless think of other sorts of measures that might be involved in physiotherapy research and it might be useful to make a list of these.

Any measurement you use belongs to one of four main categories of measurement. It is important to be able to distinguish *which* category your particular measure comes into because it will affect the sort of statistical test you can use to analyse your results — some tests can only be used with some categories of measurement.

Key concepts

When you carry out research you will be involved in measuring something. These measurements form your data or results and fall into one of four main categories of measurement. You need to be able to identify which category your own measurements come into, because this will affect the way in which you analyse your data, since some statistical tests can only be used with certain categories of measurement.

The four categories of measurement are called *levels of measurement* and each category gives us a different amount of information:

1. Nominal level or scale — the most basic level which gives us least information about the data.

2. Ordinal level or scale — the next level which provides all the information of the Nominal scale plus some additional information about the data
3. Interval level or scale — a higher level of measurement which provides all the information of the nominal *and* ordinal scales but which offers additional information about the data.
4. Ratio level or scale — the highest level of all which provides all the information of the nominal, ordinal *and* interval scales but which offers further information still about the data.

For the purposes of statistical analysis, the interval and ratio scales are combined to form a single category, and this is how we will be dealing with them in this book.

Before we go on to look at what these levels actually mean, you may find it useful to remember the mnemonic **NOIR** (as it becomes most students' 'bête noir' trying to understand which category is which) to help you with the *order* of the different levels.

NOMINAL LEVEL

Let's take the nominal level first of all. As you may have guessed, this is simply a *naming* category, in that it only gives names or labels to your data without implying any order, quality or dimension. So, for example, you might want to ascertain how many of the applicants for places at a School of Physiotherapy come from particular areas. You call one region Area A, another Area B, and another Area C and count up how many applicants fall into each category. This is a *nominal* level of measurement, because it has simply allowed you to allocate your data into one of three named categories.

Two important points are worth noting here. I have just said that this level of measurement has no implication for degree, order or quality of the data, which means that we could very easily alter the headings of the categories in any way, without affecting the results. So, for instance, Area A could just as easily have been called Area C or D, or X, Y or Z or Banana or Apple, since it will not affect the number of applicants who have come from that region.

Secondly, the categories are mutually exclusive, in that an applicant can *only* come from one area. Thus, once we have allocated a subject to one particular category, they cannot be allocated to any other category.

Let's take an example. If you were looking at the relationship of two different physiotherapy schools to final exam success, you might take

School A ⎰ and count up the number of passes
School B ⎱ and fails at each

What you are measuring here is exam success, but all you have done is to use two labels — *pass* and *fail* — and you have counted up how many students in each school achieved more than 50% (pass category) and how many achieved less (fail category). You might end up with the following data:

	Pass	Fail
School A	29	11
School B	33	7

Now, these categories pass and fail could have been called anything and it would not have affected the results. So we could have used:

Category dog = students achieving over 50%
Category cat = students achieving less than 50%

and the numbers would have been identical. Furthermore, a student who comes into the Category dog (or pass) cannot also come into the category cat (or fail) and so this sort of level of measurement involves mutually exclusive categories.

This level of measurement gives us very little information about our data. You don't know *how* well the students have passed — all School A's pass students may have achieved 90% +, while all School B's passes may have been between 50–55%. You also don't know how bad the fails are — 0% or 43% — *all* you know is that a certain number of students can be labelled 'pass' and a certain number 'fail'. Therefore, this is a nominal level of measurement — and as you can see, it doesn't tell us a great deal. For example, if you had to recommend one of these schools on the basis of nominal data, you would probably suggest School B because it achieved 33 passes to School A's 29. But if School A had average pass marks of 90% + as opposed to School B's 50–55%, you might want to change your recommendation. However, you wouldn't know this from nominal data alone, since all this category allows you to do is to classify your data under the broad headings of pass and fail.

Political opinion polls which simply categorise people into Conservative, Labour, Lib/SDP and Don't Knows are nominal scales. Voting on a particular issue in a meeting categorises people into For, Against and Abstain and so is a nominal scale. We don't know how conservative a respondent in a poll is, or how Against a voter in a meeting is — we just know that they can be allocated to a particular category.

The following are also examples of the nominal level of measurement:

a. The number of male vs female applicants for physiotherapy places at School A may be 39 males to 123 females. You don't know how masculine the male applicants are, or how good their 'A'-level results are, or how suitable they are, all you know is that you have 39 male applicants and 123 females.

b. You send a questionnaire to all the clinical physiotherapists in a district asking them to indicate:

Do you smoke?   Yes _____   No _____

You get a set of replies, which suggests that 42 people smoke, and 101 do not. But you do not know how *many* cigarettes the smokers smoke — it may be 5 per day or 65. All you know is that 42 physiotherapists in a particular district smoke and 101 do not.

Activity 16 (Answers on page 279)

Look at the following measures you might use in a piece of research, and indicate how these might be converted into a nominal category of measurement:

1. improvement in incontinence following therapy
2. reduced incidence of chest infections following breathing exercises
3. increased range of movement in a leg following manipulation
4. keeping appointments at an outpatients' clinic
5. perceptions of the quality of physiotherapy.

ORDINAL SCALE

The next category of measurement is the *ordinal scale* which tells us a bit more about our data. The ordinal scale allows us to *rank order* our data according to the dimension we are interested in, for example:

most preferred   — least preferred
most improved   — least improved
most competent — least competent.

Suppose you asked a clinical supervisor to rank order a set of students on their competence during a placement, because you wanted to see if clinical performance was related to 'A'-level grades. The supervisor may come up with the following list:

Competence position	Student
1 (Most competent)	Catherine A.
2	Jane C.
3	Jackie S.
4	Carol R.
5 (Least competent)	Susan D.

What we have is a rank ordering of these students in terms of the dimension we're interested in — their competence. We still don't have a great deal of information about them, however, because we don't know *how* much better Catherine A. is from Jane C. or how much worse Susan D. is from the rest (or in fact, whether any of them are competent at all). All we know is that Catherine A. *is* better than Jane C. who in turn *is* better than Jackie S. — but we don't know how much better. In order words, we have a *relative* and not an *absolute* measure of competence. It is also important to note that the differences between each pair of ordinal positions is not necessarily the same, i.e. the difference in competence between

Catherine A. and Jane C. may not be the same as the difference between Jane C. and Jackie S.

Another example of an ordinal scale of measurement is the use of a *point-scale*. For example, in the previous study, you might alternatively have asked the clinical supervisor to indicate on the following scale how competent each student was:

1	2	3	4	5
totally incompetent	fairly incompetent	average	quite competent	extremely competent

Here we have a dimension of most competent to least competent on a 5-point scale, and on which each student may be rated. Therefore, had we asked the clinical supervisor to assess the students using this scale, we might have found the following:

Competence score	Student
5	Catherine A.
4	Jane C.
3	Jackie S.
2	Carol R.
1	Susan D.

Again, the difference between each pair of scores must not be assumed to be the same; the difference in competence between:

$$\begin{cases} 5 \text{ (extremely competent)} \\ \text{and} \\ 4 \text{ (quite competent)} \end{cases}$$

may not be the same as between:

$$\begin{cases} 1 \text{ (totally incompetent)} \\ \text{and} \\ 2 \text{ (fairly incompetent)} \end{cases}$$

In our earlier example on the smoking questionnaire, you could modify your question from:

Do you smoke?   Yes _____   No _____ to

What sort of smoker would you classify yourself as:

1	2	3	4	5
don't smoke	light	average	quite heavy	very heavy

Again, we don't know whether the physiotherapist who selects 'very heavy' smokes 60 or 100 cigarettes a day, but we do know that she smokes more than the light smoker. Similarly, someone who scores 4 may not smoke *twice* the number of cigarettes as someone who scores 2. All we know is that someone with a score of 4 does smoke more than someone with a score of 2. We can see particularly clearly from this example how the ordinal scale tells us more information about our data than the nominal scale. If we use this rank ordering technique, we can count up the number of *non-smokers* (anyone who scores 1) and the number of *smokers* (those who score 2, 3, 4 and 5) and this gives us the information provided by the nominal scale. However, the ordinal scale adds a *dimension* to the label of 'smoker', in that it allows us to measure people according to whether they are heavy, average or light smokers. In other words, it gives us a bit more information than the nominal level.

Activity 17 (Answers on pages 279–280)

Look back at the examples given on page 78 and convert each of these to an ordinal level of measurement.

INTERVAL/RATIO LEVEL

The interval level or scale of measurement is like the ordinal scale, except that it *does* assume equal intervals in its measurement. Interval scales are measures such as percentage in an exam, range of movement etc. These measurements have two things in common. Firstly, they assume *equal* intervals, such that it is possible to say that the *difference* between scores of 30% and 60% (i.e. 30%) is *half* the difference of that between scores of 30% and 90% (i.e. 60%). Similarly, the *difference* between marks of 40% and 50% on an exam is exactly the same as the difference between 80% and 90% (i.e. 10%). If we look back to the ordinal scale of measurement, we cannot make these statements, because we simply don't know whether the difference between scores of 1 and 3 on a 5-point scale is the same as the difference between 3 and 5. In order words the gap between 'no smoker' and 'average smoker' is not necessarily identical to the gap between 'average smoker' and 'very heavy' smoker (see above).

The second point to note is that the interval scale does not have an absolute zero point although sometimes one is arbitrarily imposed. For example, even if a student scores 0 on an anatomy exam we cannot really assume she has no knowledge of anatomy — just that we did not ask what she did know. Similarly, unless circumstances are extreme, there can be no zero score for percentage range of movement. The ratio level of measurement is like the interval level except that it does have an absolute zero. It includes measures such as distance, height, weight, time etc. Do *not* worry about this point, because for the purposes of statistical tests, interval and ratio scales are treated as the same. From now on, these two levels of measurement will be collapsed to form one category, which will be referred to as the interval/ratio level.

If, then, we look back at the example of students' competence on clinical placement, our clinical supervisor could have given the students a test (marks out of 50, say), rather than rank ordering them. The results might have looked like this:

Mark	Student
44	Catherine A.
39	Jane C.
30	Jackie S.
22	Carol R.
11	Susan D.

From this data, we can see that the difference between Catherine A. and Carol R. is twice the difference between Carol R. and Susan D. In addition, from this data we could rank order the scores to find each student's position in the group (ordinal level of measurement) and also we could classify the students into pass/fail (nominal level of measurement). Therefore, the interval/ratio level of measurement gives us more information than the ordinal scale, which in turn tells us more than the nominal scale. Again, if we look at our smoking example, we could modify our questionnaire again and simply ask 'How many cigarettes do you smoke per day?' We might get a range of answers from 0 to 60, and from this, we can say that someone who smokes 60 daily, smokes twice the amount of the person who smokes 30, three times the amount of the person who smokes 20, four times the amount of the person who smokes 15, and so on. We could also:

rank order the replies from heaviest smoker to lightest
(ordinal scale)
classify the replies into smokers and non-smokers
(nominal scale)

As a result, it can be seen that the interval/ratio level of measurement gives us all the information of the nominal and ordinal levels, plus a bit more.

It should be mentioned here that sometimes researchers treat point-scales as though they were interval rather than ordinal scales, because when constructing the point-scale they have *assumed* equal intervals between the points. Sometimes this is entirely legitimate, for example, when analysing questionnaire data. As a broad rule-of-thumb, if you construct a point-scale with *at least 7 points* on it, and are assuming that the distances between the points are comparable, then you may wish to classify this as an interval scale for the purposes of analysis.

Activity 18 (Answers on pages 280–281)

1–5 Look back at the five examples given on page 78 and convert the measures to interval/ratio scores.
6 Look at the following data, and construct:
    nominal
    ordinal
    interval/ratio
    level of measurement for each one, e.g. to look at the incidence of low back pain among welders at the local car factory, you could measure:

    (i) How many had experienced low back pain and how many had not experienced low back pain over the last 2 years (nominal)

    (ii) Frequency of back pain using a 5-point scale by asking: Indicate how often you have experienced back pain over the last 2 years (ordinal):

1	2	3	4	5
never	rarely	sometimes	quite often	very often

    (iii) Frequency of back pain using absolute number of incidents (interval/ratio):

    How many times have you experienced back pain over the last 2 years?

Using the same format, construct nominal, ordinal and interval/ratio levels of measurement for the following:

    (i) accuracy of shooting an arrow at a target

    (ii) improvement in mobility after a hip replacement operation

    (iii) relief of neck and arm pain following use of a cervical collar.

7.   Look at the following measurements and say whether they are nominal, ordinal or interval/ratio:

    (i) Number of attenders vs non-attenders at an outpatients' clinic.

    (ii) Patients' ratings of the degree of confidence they have in their physiotherapist, on a 7-point scale.

    (iii) Number of work hours lost through low back pain in physiotherapists on a neurological ward.

    (iv) Percentage of knee movement regained following physiotherapy for leg fractures.

    (v) Recovery time in days following physiotherapy for cardiothoracic surgery patients.

Remember that you need to be able to distinguish between nominal, ordinal and interval/ratio levels of measurement, because the level of measurement will affect the statistical test you can use to analyse your data. More information about this will be given in Chapter 6.

Key concepts

There are four levels of measurement, each of which gives us a different amount of information about our data.

- Nominal gives us least information and simply allows our data to be labelled, e.g. pass/fail, male/female, over 60/under 60, improvement/no improvement.
- Ordinal gives us a bit more information in that it allows us to put our data into a rank order, according to the dimension we are interested in, e.g. most competent to least, heaviest smoker to lightest, greatest movement to least etc.
- Interval/ratio give us more information, in that they deal with actual numerical scores, e.g. weight, height, time, percentage, pressure, capacity etc., which allow direct mathematical comparisons to be made.

REVIEW

Let's recap on the essential guidelines involved in designing a piece of research that have been covered so far.

1. Have you formulated an experimental hypothesis which clearly predicts a relationship between two variables? Have you stated your null (no relationship) hypothesis?

2. Are you going to test this hypothesis using a correlational design (i.e., are you predicting that as scores on one variable go up, so scores on the other variable go up or down accordingly)? Or are you going to use an experimental design which will test for differences between conditions or subject groups? If you are going to use a correlational design, go on to Chapter 11.

3. If you are going to use an experimental design, have you sorted out *what* you are going to measure (i.e. what is the DV?) Have you decided *when* you will take the pre-test measures of the DV and the post-test measures? What *level* of measurement are you using?

4. Will you be using a control group?
Is this ethically acceptable? If you are not, how many experimental conditions have you decided upon?

5. Who are your subjects going to be? Can you select them randomly? How many will you need?

6. Are you going to use a different, same or matched subject design? Are you sure that this is the most appropriate design for your hypothesis? Why?
If you are going to use a matched-subject design, have you identified the critical variables on which the Ss have to be matched?

7. Is there any need to counterbalance the conditions to overcome order effects?

8. Have you controlled for experimenter bias?

9. What are the sources of constant error? Have you controlled or eliminated them? Have you taken account of the random errors as far as you are able?

10. What significance level are you going to use? Is this appropriate for your research?

6

Matching the research design to the statistical test

DECIDING WHICH STATISTICAL TEST TO USE

The previous chapters have all been concerned with how to design a piece of research to test an hypothesis. Once you have designed and carried out your research, you need to analyse your data to find out whether the results do, in fact, support your hypothesis. The analysis involves using statistical tests. However, there is no single all-purpose test which you can use to analyse your results, *since each experimental design has an appropriate statistical test*. Therefore, one of your tasks as a researcher is to match up the appropriate statistical test with your research design. If you select the wrong test to analyse your data, then your conclusions will be vitiated — it's as critical as that. Unfortunately, many people become very worried about this matching task, but as long as you ask yourself some basic questions about your design, you shouldn't have too much trouble. A word of warning first, though — when you are *planning* your research project, do ensure that you know which statistical test you will be using. All too often people carry out their experiment without doing this first and then find that they don't know how to analyse the results, or that they need a complicated computer programme which they can't get access to. So, make sure at the planning stage that you know which statistical test you will need for your design.

> **Key concept**
>
> Each experimental design has its own statistical test which *must* be used when analysing the results. Thus, a key feature when *planning* your research is to match up the design with the appropriate statistical test.

Therefore, to decide on which statistical test to use with an experimental design, the following questions must be asked:

1. Have you got an experimental or a correlational design?

To answer this, it is usually easier to look back at your hypothesis and decide whether you were predicting *differences* in your results (for example, between patient groups, types of treatment, males and females) or whether you were predicting *similarities* between sets of data. If you were predicting *differences*, you will have used an *experimental design*, while if you were predicting *similarities*, you will have used a *correlational design*. Since this is often a focus of confusion for some people, it may be useful to go over the concepts again.

If you look back to Chapter 3, you will see that in an *experimental design*, we manipulate one variable (the independent variable) and measure the effect of this on the other variable (the dependent variable). So, if you were hypothesising that clapping is more effective than breathing exercises for cystic fibrosis patients, your IV would be type of treatment and the DV would be effectiveness. Typically, you would design an experiment whereby you gave one group of patients breathing exercises and another group clapping (manipulation of the IV) and after a fixed period you would compare the progress of the two groups (you measure the effect on the DV of manipulating the IV). Here then, you would be looking for *differences* between the two groups in terms of the effectiveness of the two treatments.

On the other hand, in some hypotheses you may predict similarities between the two variables — look back to pages 47–56. These require a correlational design. In these hypotheses you arc predicting either:

a. that as scores on one variable go up, so the scores on the other variable will also go up (positive correlation)
   or
b. that as scores on one variable go up, so the scores on the other variable will go down (negative correlation).

For example, if you hypothesised that physiotherapy students who do well on theory exams also do well on their practical assessments, you would take a group of students and look at their performance in both situations, on the assumption that the *higher* the theory mark, the *higher* the corresponding practical mark. This is called a *positive correlation*.

Alternatively, you may predict a link between the amount of dietary fibre eaten daily and the incidence of diverticular disease, such that the *higher* the amount of fibre, the *lower* the corresponding incidence of diverticulitis. This is called a *negative correlation*.

In these correlational designs you do *not* manipulate one variable to see what effect it has on the other; instead you take a whole range of scores on one variable and see whether they are related to a whole range of scores on the other variable. If you are still unclear about the differences between experimental and correlational designs, re-read Chapter 3.

2. How many conditions do you have?

If you have a correlational design, you need to ask whether you are comparing two sets of results, or *more* than two sets. Once you have answered this, you need ask yourself no more questions. Turn to Chapter 11 for more information on how to analyse results from correlational designs.

If you have an experimental design, however, you need to decide how many experimental and control conditions you have (see pages 45–47) since designs with only *two* conditions in total require a different type of statistical test to those with *more* than two conditions. For example, if you compared two groups of patients, one of whom had received some treatment (experimental condition) and the other whom had received *no* treatment (control condition), then you would have two conditions. If you had compared two types of treatment (i.e. two experimental conditions) you would again have two conditions. On the other hand, if you had compared the effectiveness of three treatment procedures, you would have three conditions. Look back to page 47 to refresh your memory on this.

3. Have you got a same, matched or different subject design?

The next question is concerned with whether you used the same, matched or different subjects in your experiment. For example, did you use just *one* group of subjects for all conditions (e.g. comparing the attitudes of one group of physiotherapists to paraplegic vs hemiplegic patients). Or did you use two or more totally different groups of subjects and compare them in some way (e.g. a comparison of attendance levels at an outpatients' department of Asian vs West Indian patients?) Or did you use two or more groups of subjects who were matched on certain key features (e.g. a comparison of the quality of newly qualified physiotherapists from three different training schools, which would necessitate matching the subjects on such variables as 'A'-level grades, attendance levels etc.) (see Ch. 4).

Remember, for the purposes of statistical analysis, matched and same subject designs are treated alike, so you only have to decide between:

same/matched subject design

or

different subject design

These questions can be set out as a decision chart like the one on pages 90–95.

(Note that the names of the appropriate statistical tests are given in the boxes on the chart.) You can see from this chart that sometimes the names of two or three tests are given. This does *not* mean that any one of them can be selected but that instead each requires slightly different conditions for use, for example, a different level of measurement. These differences are outlined in the relevant chapter. You will also notice that you are given the choice of *non-parametric* or *parametric* tests. The differences between these will be outlined before proceeding to the decision charts.

Key concepts

Every experimental design has its own statistical test(s) which *must* be used to analyse the data. In order to select the appropriate statistical test for your own design you must ask yourself a number of questions:

1. Were you looking for differences (i.e. an experimental design) or similarities (i.e. a correlational design).
   If you had an experimental design, then you must also ask:
2. How many conditions were there?
   (Two or more than two)
3. Did you use the same or matched subjects in each condition?
   Or did you use different subjects in each condition?

PARAMETRIC AND NON-PARAMETRIC TESTS

You will notice that in the boxes with the names of the statistical tests, on pages 90–95 there are the headings 'Parametric Test' and 'Non-Parametric Test'. Essentially, for most of the designs you are likely to use, you have a choice of using a *parametric* test or a *non-parametric* test. What is the difference?

Basically, a parametric test is a much more sensitive tool of statistical analysis. If, for example, you are comparing responses to two different kinds of treatment, and there *are* differences in responsiveness, the parametric test is more likely to find them than is the non-parametric test. Perhaps the point can be clarified by an analogy. Supposing you were making a cake and you wanted to weigh out the ingredients. You have two weighing machines in the house — the bathroom scales and the kitchen scales. You *could* use your bathroom scales to weigh out your 8 oz of sugar, but they will give you a less accurate and less sensitive reading than your kitchen scales. The non-parametric test is like the bathroom scales as it *will* analyse your results but it will not be as fine or as sensitive as the analysis of the parametric test — the kitchen scales.

If parametric tests are so good, then why do we bother with non-parametric tests at all? Like most things that are good, there are prices to pay and conditions to fulfil, and so it is with parametric tests. Before you can use one to analyse your results, four conditions have to be satisfied. The first of these is critical — your data *must* be of an interval/ratio level of measurement, since parametric tests *cannot* be used on nominal or ordinal data. This condition *cannot ever* be violated. The other three conditions are not quite as important, and may be waived to some degree. The first of these is that your subjects should be randomly selected from the population they represent. Second, your data should be normally distributed. As you will probably remember from Chapter 2 a normal distribution looks like an inverted U shape and you can plot your data on a graph to find out whether it is (more or less) normally distributed. Third, the variation in the results from each condition should be roughly the same. This means that the *range* of scores in each condition should be more or less similar. If, for instance, the scores in one condition ranged from 20–120, while for the other they ranged from 60–80, the degree of variation in each condition's scores would be too dissimilar for a parametric test to be used. On the other hand if they ranged from 50–100 in one condition and 60–90 in the other, this would be acceptable. To each of these three conditions we would add the caveat 'within reason', because parametric tests are said to be 'robust'. Essentially, what this means is that it does not matter too much if you cannot fulfil the last three conditions; as long as your data is of an interval/ratio level, and there are no glaring deviations with respect to the other three conditions, you can use a parametric test.

The following table may help to clarify this point:

Level of measurement	Type of test which can be used
Nominal	Non-parametric
Ordinal	Non-parametric
Interval	Parametric and non-parametric
Ratio	Parametric and non-parametric

If you're ever in doubt as to whether you've satisfied the conditions adequately, then use a non-parametric test, since this is an error to caution. *So, when in doubt, use the non-parametric test.*

Key concepts

The results from any research design may usually be analysed either by a parametric or a non-parametric test. A parametric test is much more sensitive and will identify significant results more readily than a non-parametric test. However, before you can use a parametric test, four conditions must be fulfilled:

- the data must be on an interval/ratio level
- the subjects should have been randomly selected
- the data should be normally distributed
- the variance in the results from each condition should be similar.

The first condition is essential.
The other three can be violated to some extent.
Non-parametric tests do not require these conditions to be fulfilled and can be used with any level of measurement.

Table 6.1A

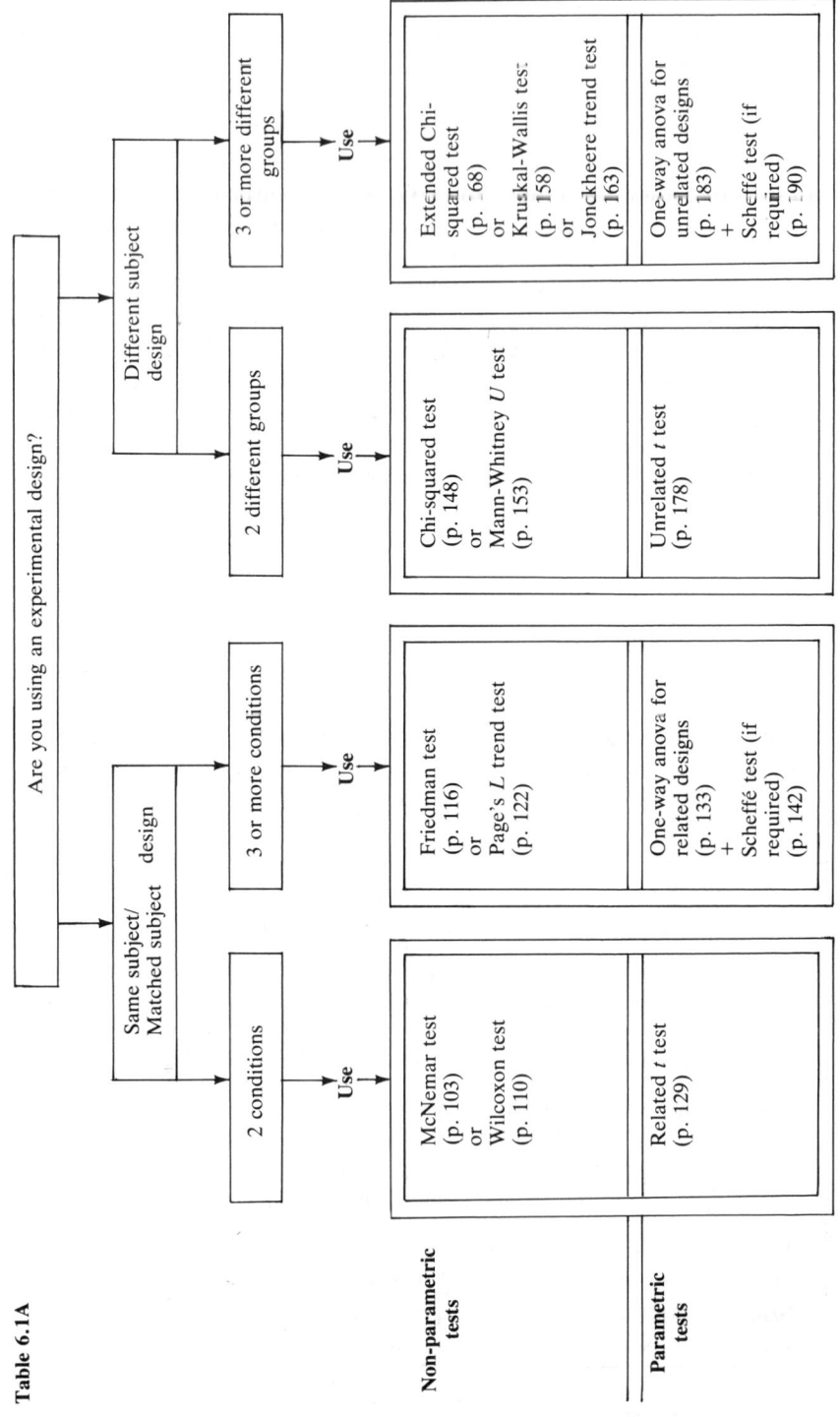

Are you using an experimental design?

Same subject/Matched subject design

Different subject design

2 conditions

3 or more conditions

2 different groups

3 or more different groups

Use

Non-parametric tests

McNemar test (p. 103) or Wilcoxon test (p. 110)

Friedman test (p. 116) or Page's *L* trend test (p. 122)

Chi-squared test (p. 148) or Mann-Whitney *U* test (p. 153)

Extended Chi-squared test (p. 168) or Kruskal-Wallis test (p. 158) or Jonckheere trend test (p. 163)

Parametric tests

Related *t* test (p. 129)

One-way anova for related designs (p. 133) + Scheffé test (if required) (p. 142)

Unrelated *t* test (p. 178)

One-way anova for unrelated designs (p. 183) + Scheffé test (if required) (p. 190)

Table 6.1B

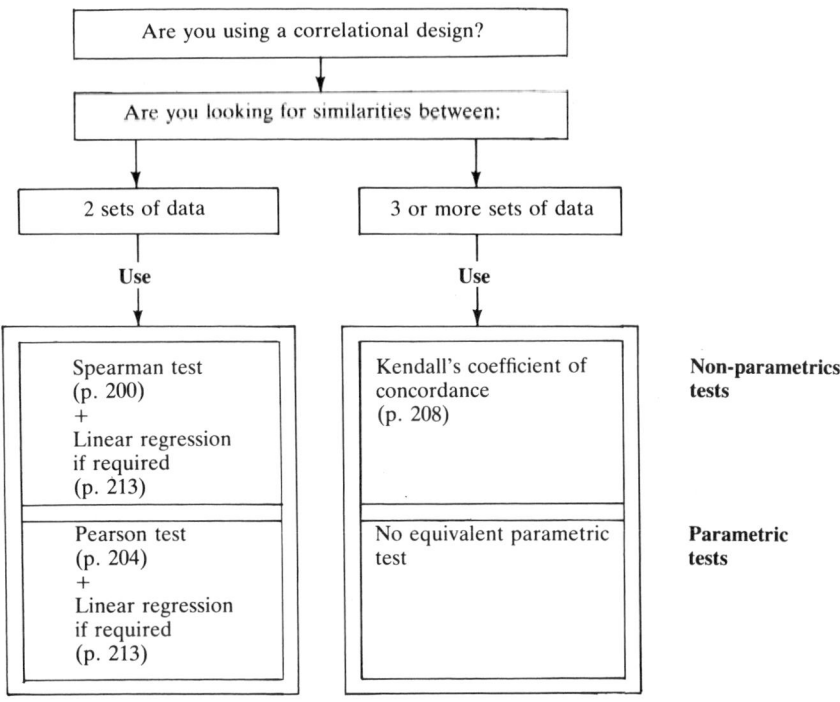

Alternatively, some students prefer to make this decision by using diagrammatic representations of the design. These are set out below, together with some examples.

EXPERIMENTAL DESIGNS

Same subject designs		Test	
		Non-parametric	Parametric

Example 1

One group of Ss — takes part in *Condition 1* / takes part in *Condition 2* } Compared for differences between conditions

McNemar test (if data is nominal) or Wilcoxon (if data is other than nominal) — Non-parametric

Related *T* test (if data is interval/ratio) — Parametric

H_1 Elderly patients develop more rapport with uniformed physiotherapists than with non-uniformed physiotherapists.

Method Select a group of elderly patients and measure rapport (a) with uniformed physiotherapists and (b) with non-uniformed physiotherapists, i.e. *one* group of patients measured under both conditions.

Same subject designs		Test	
		Non-parametric	Parametric

Example 2

One group of Ss takes part in *Condition 1* / takes part in *Condition 2* / takes part in *Condition 3* (etc.) ⎫ Compared for differences between conditions ⎬

Non-parametric	Parametric
Friedman or Page's *L* trend (If data is other than nominal)	One-way anova for related designs (if data is interval/ratio) + Scheffé test if required

H₁ The attitudes of a group of physiotherapists to 3 (or more) types of patient differ significantly.

Method Select a group of physiotherapists and measure their attitudes to 3 types of patient, i.e. *one* group of physios measured under 3 different conditions.

[It can be seen that this design is an extension of Example 1.]

Different subject designs		Test	
		Non-parametric	Parametric

Example 3

Subject Group 1 takes part in *Condition 1* ⎫ Compared for differences between conditions ⎬

Subject Group 2 takes part in *Condition 2*

Non-parametric	Parametric
Chi-squared test (if data is nominal) or Mann-Whitney *U* test (if data is other than nominal)	Unrelated *t* test (if data is interval/ratio)

H₁ Men are more likely to experience respiratory complications following cardiothoracic surgery than are women.

Method Select a group of male cardiothoracic patients and a group of female cardiothoracic patients and compare degree of respiratory complications, i.e. two different groups of Ss compared.

Example 4

Subject Group 1 takes part in *Condition 1* ⎫
Subject Group 2 takes part in *Condition 2* ⎬ Compared for differences between conditions
Subject Group 3 (etc.) takes part in *Condition 3* ⎭

Non-parametric	Parametric
Extended Chi-squared test (if data is nominal) or Kruskal-Wallis or Jonckheere trend (if data is other than nominal)	One-way anova for unrelated designs (if data is interval/ratio) + Scheffé test if required

H₁ There is a difference in responsiveness to interferential treatment of middle-age stress incontinence in women with no children, 2 children or 4+ children.

Method Select 3 groups of women: 1 with no children, 1 with 2 children and 1 with 4 or more children and compare their responsiveness to treatment, i.e. 3 different groups of Ss compared

[This is an extension of Example 3 above.]

Matched subject designs		Test	
		Non-parametric	Parametric

Example 5

Subjects matched on certain key variables {

Subject Group 1 takes part in *Condition 1*

Subject Group 2 takes part in *Condition 2*

	Non-parametric	Parametric
Compared for differences between conditions	McNemar (if data is nominal) or Wilcoxon (if data is other than nominal)	Related *t* test (if data is interval/ratio)

H_1 Cast bracing is more effective than traction in the treatment of leg fractures.

Method Take two groups of leg fracture patients, matched on key variables such as age, sex, prior fractures, and fitness and treat one group with traction and the other with cast bracing. Compare their progress,
i.e. two groups of Ss *matched* on certain critical factors, and compared for progress.

Example 6

Subjects matched on certain key variables {

Subject Group 1 takes part in *Condition 1*

Subject Group 2 takes part in *Condition 2*

Subject Group 3 (etc.) takes part in *Condition 3*

	Non-parametric	Parametric
Compared for differences between conditions	Friedman or Page's *L* trend (if data is other than nominal)	One-way anova for related designs (if data is interval/ratio) + Scheffé test if required

H_1 To extend the above hypothesis, you add a further treatment group which uses plaster of Paris.

Method You select a further group of leg fracture patients matched with groups 1 and 2 on age, sex, prior fractures and fitness and compare the progress of the 3 groups,
i.e. 3 groups of Ss *matched* on certain critical factors, and compared for progress.

You should note that in Examples 2, 4 and 6, you can use more than 3 groups or conditions and still apply the same test.

CORRELATIONAL DESIGNS

Design	Test	
	Non-parametric	Parametric

Example 7

These may predict:

a. positive correlation, i.e. *high* scores on one variable are associated with *high* scores on the other

Spearman (if data is other than nominal) + Linear regression if required

Pearson (if data is interval/ratio) + Linear regression if required

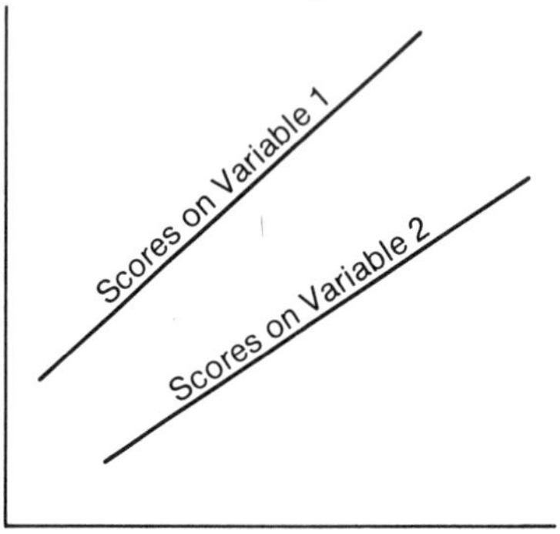

Fig. 28

H₁ There is a correlation between age and recovery time following gall bladder removal, such that the *older* the patient, the *longer* the recovery time.

Method Select a whole age range of cholecystectomy patients and note their recovery time from operation to discharge.

b. negative correlation, i.e. *high* scores on one variable are related to *low* scores on the other.

Spearman (if data is other than nominal) + Linear regression if required

Pearson (if data is interval/ratio) + Linear regression if required

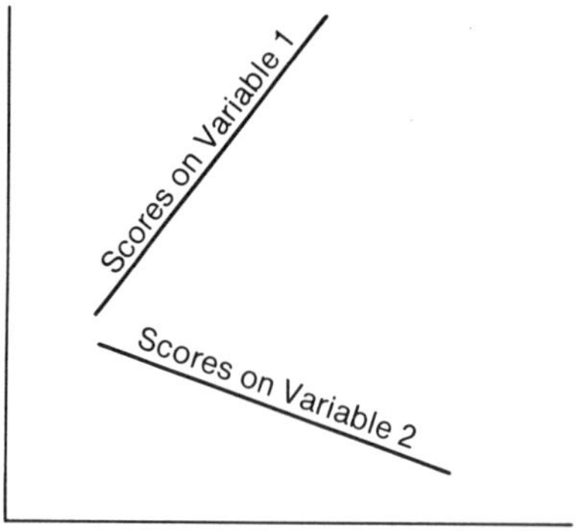

Fig. 29

H₁ There is a correlation between vital capacity and number of cigarettes smoked, with *high* numbers of cigarettes being associated with *low* vital capacity.

Method Select a whole range of smokers (e.g. non-smokers to 80+ per day and measure their vital capacity).

Design	Test	
	Non-parametric	Parametric

Example 8
Where you are looking for the degree of similarity between *3 or more* sets of scores:

Kendall coefficient of concordance (if data is other than nominal)

There is no parametric test

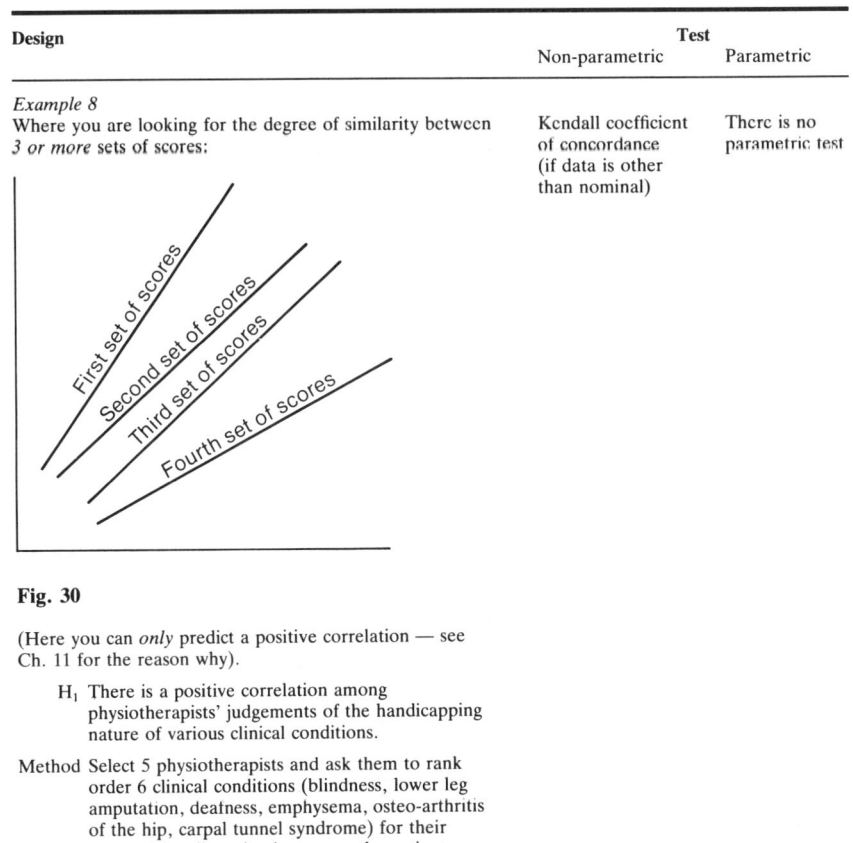

Fig. 30

(Here you can *only* predict a positive correlation — see Ch. 11 for the reason why).

 H₁ There is a positive correlation among physiotherapists' judgements of the handicapping nature of various clinical conditions.

Method Select 5 physiotherapists and ask them to rank order 6 clinical conditions (blindness, lower leg amputation, deafness, emphysema, osteo-arthritis of the hip, carpal tunnel syndrome) for their assumed handicapping impact on the patient.

Activity 19 (Answers on page 281)

Look at the following brief descriptions of some research projects, and decide which statistical tests you should use. (Quote both the parametric and non-parametric alternatives where relevant, since at this stage you would not know whether your data would allow you to use a parametric test.)

1. In order to compare the speciality preferences of a group of newly-qualified physiotherapists and a group of senior physiotherapists you select two groups of 30 subjects to represent each group and ask them to state whether they prefer geriatric or paediatric work.
2. To find out whether leg fracture patients progress faster on hydrotherapy or suspension, you select two groups of 15 Ss, matched on certain key features such as age, sex, prior fractures etc. and compare their progress after 4 weeks' treatment.
3. On the assumption that seniority in the physiotherapy profession is related to high absenteeism rates, as a result of stress, (the higher the grade, the greater the absenteeism) you look at the number of days off taken by all grades of physiotherapist at a large general hospital.
4. To find out whether social class is related to compliance with exercise regimes following laminectomy operations, you select 30 patients from social classes 1

and 2 and 30 from social classes 4 and 5 and compare their reported compliance, on a 5-point scale.
5. To compare the effectiveness of three types of walking aid for hip replacement patients, you select three groups of Ss, matched on key variables, such as age, fitness etc, and give one group Zimmer frames, the second group walking sticks and the third group crutches. Their mobility after 3 weeks is compared.
6. In order to compare the attitudes of three different grades of physiotherapist to a new set of shift hours, you select a group of 15 superintendent physios, 15 senior IIs and 15 basic grades and compare their attitudes, using a point scale.

LOOKING UP THE RESULTS OF YOUR ANALYSIS IN THE PROBABILITY TABLES

Let's suppose you have designed and carried out your experiments and have analysed the results using the correct statistical test. As you will remember, it was stated earlier that a statistical test will give you a result which you look up in a set of probability tables in order to find out whether your results are significant and support your hypothesis. This process will be described more fully in the chapters which deal with the particular statistical tests, but an outline of the general principles will be given here.

Each statistical test will provide you with a value or figure for an alphabetic letter which you look up in a set of probability tables *for that particular test*. It is important to note that each statistical test has its own set of probability tables, which you will find at the back of this book. Thus, the Mann-Whitney U-test will provide you with a value of U which is looked up in the probability tables for the Mann-Whitney test (see Tables A2.7a–d). The Wilcoxon test provides you with a value of T which is looked up in the probability tables for the Wilcoxon test, and so on. More details on this will be given with the description for each statistical test.

However, before you can look up that numerical value, some tests require an additional numerical value — either the number of Ss you used or a number called the degrees of freedom (df). This concept which is quite a complex one to understand refers to the degree of potential variability in the data. [The reader is referred to Ferguson (1976) for a discussion of this.] However, although the concept is hard to understand, the df is very easy to calculate. The details of how to do this will be given in the description of the tests which require the df.

However, before you can conclude whether your numerical value represents a significant result from your experiment, you require one further piece of information — namely whether you have a one- or two-tailed hypothesis.

ONE- AND TWO-TAILED HYPOTHESES

The way in which you state your hypothesis has implications for how you look up your numerical value in the probability tables. Some hypotheses are stated very specifically in that they predict *precisely* what the results will be. For example, if the hypothesis was 'Elderly patients experience more rapport with uniformed rather than non-uniformed physios', we are predicting a very *precise* outcome in that we are saying that the patients will experience *more* rapport with *uniformed* physios. Again, if we hypothesised that 'leg fractures improve faster with traction than with cast bracing' we are making a precise prediction, because we are assuming *faster* progress with *traction*. These are known as one-tailed hypotheses or tests because the results are expected to go in *one particular direction*. The following are all examples of one-tailed hypotheses:

1. Women are *more* likely to experience complications following chole-cystectomy operations than are men.
2. Ultrasound is *more* effective than short wave diathermy for arthritic toe joints.
3. Social classes 4 and 5 are *less* likely to keep to exercise regimes than are social classes 1 and 2.
4. Children with lower leg amputations are *less* likely to suffer from negative body image than adolescents with lower leg amputations.
5. Male physiotherapy students are *more* likely to fail the clinical assessment than are females.

However, hypotheses can be stated much more vaguely, without any *precise* predictions. For example, it might have been hypothesised that elderly patients experience *different* degrees of rapport with uniformed and non-uniformed physiotherapists. In contrast to the one-tailed hypothesis which predicted *more* rapport with *uniformed* physiotherapists, this hypothesis allows for the possibility that more rapport could be experienced with *either* uniformed *or* non-uniformed physiotherapists, because it simply predicts *differences* in rapport, without specifying what these differences might be. Similarly, if we predict that leg fractures respond differently to traction and cast bracing, we are not specifying *how* they respond, but simply that there is a difference in response, which could mean leg fractures improve more with cast bracing *or* with traction. These hypotheses are known as two-tailed hypotheses or tests because the results could go in *either* of *two* directions. The following are examples of two-tailed hypotheses:

1. Senior and basic grade physiotherapists *differ* in their absenteeism rates as a result of stress.
2. Student physiotherapists with 'A'-level physics *differ* in their theory exam. performance from students without 'A'-level physics.
3. Interferential and exercise techniques are *differentially* effective in treating stress incontinence.
4. Zimmer frames and walking sticks afford *different* degrees of mobility for patients with ankylosing spondylitis.
5. Patients who are given pre-op. respiratory exercises *differ* in their inci-

dence of post op. complications from patients who are given no pre-op. respiratory exercises.

Activity 20 (Answers on pages 281–282)

Look at the following hypotheses and identify which are one-tailed and which are two-tailed:

1. Praise is a more effective motivator for mobilising exercises, when used in group rather than 1–1 situations.
2. Paraffin wax and hot soaks are differentially effective as a preparation for mobilising exercises in post-fracture patients.
3. Patients who attend for rigorous exercise regimes in back schools make fewer complaints following treatment, than patients who attend for heat treatment.
4. There is a difference in the strength of muscle contraction of a selected muscle group when preceded by 2 minutes infrared radiation as opposed to 2 minutes specific warm-up.
5. The application of lumbar traction diminishes vital capacity.

Look back at the examples of one-tailed hypotheses and convert them to two-tailed hypotheses.

Then look at the examples of two-tailed hypotheses and convert them to one-tailed hypotheses. (It does not matter in which direction you predict the results will go.)

Why is this important? Supposing you had stated a one-tailed hypothesis, (i.e. that your results will go in *one* specific direction) and having done your experiment and statistics, had ended up with a p value of 1%. This means that there is a $\frac{1}{100}$ chance that your results are due to random error. However, had your hypothesis been two-tailed instead, you would be predicting that your results could go in either of *two* directions. Therefore, because your results could go in either of *two* directions there will be *twice* the possibility that random error could account for your results and so for exactly the same data your p value would be doubled to 2%, i.e. a $\frac{2}{100}$ chance that your results are due to random error. Let's illustrate this with an example.

Suppose you had hypothesised that exercise is *more* effective than clapping for increasing lung capacity in cystic fibrosis patients (i.e. you have stated a one-tailed hypothesis), you would probably have selected two groups of patients, one of which received exercise and the other clapping. You would expect that the lung capacities of the exercise group following treatment would be generally larger. Suppose again, that your results suggest this is the case, and you end up with a p value of 5%. This means that there is a $\frac{5}{100}$ chance that your results are due to error, and that for every 100 patients treated in this way, 5 would not improve significantly as a result of treatment. However, had you simply hypothesised that clapping and exercise are *differentially* effective in increasing lung capacity then you would expect *either* the exercise group *or* the clapping group to do better. Your results would be the same as those above (only your hypothesis has changed), but your p value would be 10% (i.e. doubled) because if your results are expected to go in either of *two* directions, there must be *twice* the possibility that random error can account for the results. Let's see how this works in practice by turning to Table A2.2 (Wilcoxon).

At the top of the table you will see two headings: Level of significance for one-tailed test and Level of significance for two-tailed test. You can see that every level of significance for a two-tailed test is *twice* the corresponding level for a one-tailed test, i.e. 0.10 is twice 0.05 (above); 0.05 is twice 0.025; 0.02 is twice 0.01; 0.01 is twice 0.005.

Many students ask how they should decide on whether an hypothesis should be one or two-tailed. The answer to this lies in the background theory associated with the research you are carrying out. For example, if you are concerned with the relationship between smoking and bronchitis, the background reading that you will have done prior to embarking on this research will probably have revealed that:

a. smoking is related to *lung cancer*
b. bronchitis is associated with particular atmospheric pollution

and therefore, it would be reasonable to predict that heavy smokers are *more* likely to get bronchitis (i.e. a specific one-tailed prediction). Thus, the existing research and literature will guide your prediction here.

If, however, you were interested in looking at the effects of wearing uniform on patients' feelings, you may well have found background literature which suggests that some patients are more comfortable with uniformed physiotherapists, while others prefer the informality of the physiotherapist in 'civvies'. Thus, because the background research is less clear cut here, you would probably not wish to make a specific prediction about patients' attitudes to uniformed vs non-uniformed physiotherapists, and would therefore formulate a two-tailed hypothesis. In other words, existing research knowledge and theory should guide you when making predictions in the hypothesis.

Key concepts

When you use a statistical test to analyse the results from your research you will end up with a numerical value.

This value is looked up in the set of probability tables which are specific to the statistical test you have used. In order to look up the value you will also need to know *either* the df value *or* the number of subjects who participated in the experiment — each statistical test requires one or the other. Additionally, you must decide whether your hypothesis is one-tailed (predicts that the results will go in one direction only) or two-tailed (predicts that the results will go in either of two directions). Hypotheses which are two-tailed have *twice* the probability that random error can account for the results, and so will affect the p value for your data.

contd overleaf

Using these two values, you will end up with a p value, i.e. percentage probability that your results are due to random error. According to the size of the p value you can either claim your results are significant (i.e. support your hypothesis) or not significant (do not support your hypothesis.)

7

Non-parametric tests for same and matched subject designs

As was mentioned in the last chapter, the results from most of the designs you are likely to use can be analysed either by a non-parametric *or* a parametric statistical test. Each test does essentially the same job, but the parametric test is rather more sensitive. However, in order to use a parametric test, certain pre-requisite conditions have to be fulfilled (see Ch. 6). If you cannot fulfil these or if you have any doubts then you should use the equivalent non-parametric test. All the tests in this chapter are non-parametric ones for same and matched subject designs. In the next chapter, the equivalent parametric tests for the same designs will be covered.

So, the statistical tests covered in this chapter are appropriate for any experimental design which involves *either* one group of subjects which is used in *all* the conditions (same subject design) or alternatively two or more groups of subjects each of which is used in one condition only, but *who are matched on certain key variables* (matched subject design). (Have a look back to the examples given on pages 91 93 in the previous chapter.) Therefore, the sort of designs we are talking about are:

1. One group of subjects used in all the conditions (same subject design)

a. Two conditions

1 group of subjects — takes part in → *Condition 1*
— takes part in → *Condition 2*

Results from conditions compared for differences

or

b. *Three or more conditions*

1 group

of subjects

takes part in → Condition 1

takes part in — Condition 2

takes Part in → Condition 3
        (etc.)

Results from conditions compared for differences

2. Two or more groups of matched subjects, each of which is used in one condition only (matched subject designs)

a. *Two matched groups only*

Matched on certain Key variables {

Subject group 1 $\dfrac{takes}{part\ in}$ Condition 1

Subject group 2 $\dfrac{takes}{part\ in}$ Condition 2

Results from conditions compared for differences

or

b. *Three or more matched groups*

Matched on certain Key variables {

Subject group 1 $\dfrac{takes}{part\ in}$ Condition 1

Subject group 2 $\dfrac{takes}{part\ in}$ Condition 2

Subject group 3 $\dfrac{takes}{part\ in}$ Condition 3
(and so on)

Results from conditions compared for differences

The designs which involve *one* group doing *two* conditions (Design la) or *two matched* groups doing one condition each (Design 2a) are analysed using the McNemar test if the data is only nominal, or the Wilcoxon test if the data is ordinal or interval/ratio. The designs which involve *one* group doing *three* or more conditions (Design 1b) or 3 (or more) matched groups doing one condition each (Design 2b) are analysed using either the Friedman test or the Page's *L* trend test. Pages 116–123 will explain which of those two you should select, since each one requires slightly different conditions.

Table 7.1 Non-parametric tests for related and matched subject designs

Design	Non-Parametric test
1. One group of Ss taking part in two conditions. Results from conditions compared for differences.	McNemar test if the data is *nominal* or Wilcoxon test if the data is *ordinal or interval/ratio*.
2. Two groups of matched Ss each taking part in one condition only. Results from conditions compared for differences.	McNemar test if the data is *nominal* or Wilcoxon test if the data is *ordinal or interval/ratio*.
3. One group of Ss taking part in three or more conditions. Results from conditions compared for differences.	Friedman test or Page's *L* trend test (see pp. 116–123 for which one to use). Both these can be used with ordinal or interval/ratio data.
4. Three or more groups of *matched* Ss, each taking part in one condition only. Results from conditions compared for differences.	Friedman test or Page's *L* trend test (see pp. 116–123 for which one to use). Both these can be used with ordinal or interval/ratio data.

NON-PARAMETRIC STATISTICAL TEST FOR USE WITH SAME OR MATCHED SUBJECT DESIGNS, TWO CONDITIONS AND NOMINAL DATA

McNemar test for the significance of changes

Just to remind you, this test is used when *either* you have *one* group of subjects who are measured or tested on *two* conditions (a same subject design) and the two sets of results are then compared for any differences between them; *or* when you compare *two* groups of subjects who are *matched* on all the critical variables which might influence the results (i.e. a matched group design). Each group is tested in one condition and the results are compared for differences between them. In other words you would use this test if you had either experimental Design 1a or 2a on pages 101–102.

The McNemar test is particularly suitable for 'before and after' type situations. However, there is one very important feature of this test — it is used with *nominal* data — that is, a level of measurement which simply allows you to allocate people or responses to named categories. Essentially what the McNemar test does is to record the changes from one category to the other, across the two conditions, to see if these changes are significant. When you calculate the McNemar test, you find a numerical value for χ^2, which you then look up in Table A2.1 to see if this figure represents significant differences between the two conditions or the two matched groups.

Example

Let's imagine you've noticed over the years the degree of fear most women experience prior to having a hysterectomy. It occurs to you that a pre-op. talk to explain what will happen, and to allow them to express any doubts or anxieties may go a long way towards reducing their tension. You decide to try this and see whether your hunch is correct.

Your experimental hypothesis is:

H_1 A pre-operative talk and counselling session will reduce fear levels in hysterectomy patients

(What would your null hypothesis be?)

You select 20 pre-hysterectomy patients and note whether they are frightened about the operation.

You classify them as either

    1. little or no anxiety

       or

    2. high anxiety.

This is *nominal* data because you are simply allocating patients' responses to a named category. You then spend some time explaining to the patients what will happen, discussing any issues and problems they have etc. Following this session, the patients are asked whether their anxiety levels have reduced. According to their response, you again allocate them to one of the categories, as before.

You therefore have the following design:

1 group of 20 hysterectomy patients

takes part in → *Condition 1* Classified *before* the pre-op. talk

takes part in → *Condition 2* Classified *after* the pre-op. talk

Changes in classification compared to see if there are significant differences between the two conditions

You obtain the following results:
$\emptyset$ = Little or no anxiety
X = High anxiety

Patient	Before talk	After talk
1	$\emptyset$	$\emptyset$
2	X	$\emptyset$
3	X	$\emptyset$
4	$\emptyset$	$\emptyset$
5	X	X
6	X	$\emptyset$
7	X	X
8	$\emptyset$	$\emptyset$
9	X	$\emptyset$
10	X	$\emptyset$
11	X	X
12	X	$\emptyset$
13	$\emptyset$	$\emptyset$
14	$\emptyset$	$\emptyset$
15	$\emptyset$	$\emptyset$
16	X	X
17	X	$\emptyset$
18	X	$\emptyset$
19	X	$\emptyset$
20	X	$\emptyset$

Calculating the McNemar test

1. You must first of all record the changes that occurred from one testing to the other. In other words you must count up:

   a. how many patients changed from 'little or no anxiety' to 'high anxiety' as a result of the talk, i.e. from '$\emptyset$' before the talk to 'X' after. In the above example there are no changes of this kind.
   b. how many patients *continued* to experience very little or no anxiety after the talk, i.e. were '$\emptyset$' before the talk and '$\emptyset$' afterwards. In this example, there are 6 such patients.
   c. how many patients *continued* to experience high anxiety after the talk, i.e. were 'X' before and 'X' after. Here there were 4 such patients.
   d. how many patients changed from feeling high anxiety before the talk to feeling little or no anxiety after, i.e. changes from 'X' before the talk to '$\emptyset$' afterwards. Here there are 10.

2. These figures now have to be put in a table like the following:

After the talk

		X	$\emptyset$
	$\emptyset$	Cell A	Cell B
Before the talk			
	X	Cell C	Cell D

Cell A represents those patients who changed from $\emptyset$ to X (little anxiety to high anxiety, i.e. 0). This is calculation (a) above.

Cell B represents those patients who continued to experience little or no anxiety (stayed at $\emptyset$, i.e. 6). This is calculation (b) above.

Cell C represents those patients who continued to feel high anxiety (stayed at X, i.e. 4). This is calculation (c) above.

Cell D represents those patients who changed from high anxiety to low anxiety (changed from X to $\emptyset$, i.e. 10). This is calculation (d) above.

So, if we enter these figures into the cells, the table looks like this:

After the talk

		X	$\emptyset$
	$\emptyset$	0	6
Before the talk			
	X	4	10

Remember! You *must* organise your cells in the way indicated above, otherwise your calculations will be incorrect. In other words, which ever category is on the left-hand cell for the 'After' condition, the other category should be at the top for the 'Before' condition. The numbers in the cells should add up to the same as the number of patients tested. In this case, the number is 20.

3. Find the value of χ^2 from the formula:

$$\chi^2 = \frac{([A - D] - 1)^2}{A + D}$$

where A = the value in cell A (i.e. 0)
       D = the value in cell D (i.e. 10)

If we substitute our figures we get:

$$\chi^2 = \frac{([0 - 10^*] - 1)^2}{10}$$
$$= \frac{(9)^2}{10}$$
$$= \frac{81}{10}$$
$$\therefore \chi^2 = 8.1$$

(*If you get a minus figure in the square brackets, ignore it; i.e. –10 becomes 10)

4. Before looking up the results to see if they represent a significant change in fear, you need a further value: the df value. In the McNemar test, it is always 1.

Looking up the value of χ^2 for significance

To see whether this value of 8.1 represents a significance difference in fear levels, turn to Table A2.1, which is the probability table associated with the McNemar test (and the Chi-squared or χ^2 test — see later). Down the left-hand column you will see df values from 1 to 30. To their right are 5 numbers, called *critical values* of χ^2. To find out whether our χ^2 value is significant, look down the df column until you find our df value of 1. To the right you will see 5 critical values:

2.71   3.84   5.41   6.64   10.83

Each of these figures is associated with the probability value at the top of its column. For example, the critical vlaue of 2.71 is associated with a probability value of 0.10, for a two-tailed test. You will notice that this table only refers to two-tailed hypotheses. Where you have a one-tailed hypothesis, look up the results in the way outlined, and simply *halve* the p value (see pp 96–100).

For our χ^2 value to be significant, it has to be *equal to* or *larger* than one of the critical values to the right of df = 1. Our χ^2 value of 8.1 is larger than 2.71, 3.84, 5.41 and 6.64. We therefore take the value of 6.64 which is associated with a probability value of 0.01 for a two-tailed hypothesis, and therefore 0.005 for a one-tailed hypothesis (i.e. *half* 0.01). If you look back to our hypothesis, you will see that we are predicting a specific direction to our results, i.e. pre-operative counselling will reduce fear levels; therefore, our hypothesis is one-tailed. Now to be significant *exactly* at the 0.005 level, our χ^2 value must *equal* 6.64. Our χ^2 value is *larger* than 6.64, so that means that the probability of our results being due to random error is even *less than* 0.005. This is expressed as:

$p < 0.005$ ($<$ means 'less than')

Had our χ^2 value been exactly 6.64 we would have expressed this as:

$p = 0.005$.

Interpreting the results

Our results are associated with a probability of less than 0.005 or 0.5%. This means there is less than 0.5% chance of the results being due to random error. If you remember, a p value of 5% or less was a standard cut-off point for claiming results to be significant. As 0.5% is less than 5% our results *are* significant. However, before going on to explain what this means, you must check that the changes in fear are in the direction you predicted, that is

<table>
<tr><td>high fear</td><td></td><td>low fear</td></tr>
<tr><td>before the</td><td>changed to</td><td>after the</td></tr>
<tr><td>talk</td><td></td><td>talk</td></tr>
</table>

It is not uncommon to get significant results which are in the opposite direction to those predicted. In this case it would mean

<table>
<tr><td>low fear</td><td></td><td>high fear</td></tr>
<tr><td>before the</td><td>changed to</td><td>after the</td></tr>
<tr><td>talk</td><td></td><td>talk</td></tr>
</table>

These results, while significant, would not support your hypothesis.

If you look at the data in the table, you will see that the changes are in the predicted direction, and we can

> reject the null (no relationship)
>   hypothesis
>   and
> accept the experimental hypothesis.

We can state this in the following way:

Using a McNemar test on the data ($\chi^2 = 8.1$, df $= 1$), the results were found to be significant at $p < 0.005$ for a one-tailed test. This suggests that pre-operative counselling sessions significantly reduce the fear of hysterectomy patients.

It is very important to note, though, that there should be significant numbers involved to compute the McNemar test. If $\dfrac{\text{Cell A} + \text{Cell D}}{2}$ comes to less than 5, you cannot use the McNemar. In such a case, it would be worth your while to collect sufficient data to satisfy the above requirement.

Activity 21 (Answers on page 282)

1. To practise looking up χ^2 values for the McNemar test, look up the following and say whether you would classify them as significant.

   (i) $\chi^2 = 3.98$ df = 1   one-tailed P
   (ii) $\chi^2 = 6.71$ df = 1   one-tailed P
   (iii) $\chi^2 = 5.41$ df = 1   two-tailed P
   (iv) $\chi^2 = 2.59$ df = 1   one-tailed P
   (v) $\chi^2 = 10.96$ df = 1   two-tailed P
   (vi) $\chi^2 = 4.82$ df = 1   two-tailed P

2. Calculate a McNemar test on the following data:
   As a district physiotherapist, you wish to alter the 'on-call' duty rotas, but have so far met with opposition from the physiotherapists in the district. In fact on the last poll, only 5 out of 30 were prepared to alter their duties. You decide to send round an explanatory fact sheet, in the hope that presenting the reasons for your change might alter their views. At the end of the fact sheet you simply ask the physios to indicate whether or not they would accommodate the altered duties.
   Your hypothesis is:

H_1 Providing extra information about the reasons for changing on-call duty hours will modify the opinions of the recipients.

You obtain the following results:
$\sqrt{}$ For the change
X Against the change

Physiotherapist	Opinions prior to receipt of factsheet	Opinions after the receipt of factsheet
1	X	$\sqrt{}$
2	X	$\sqrt{}$
3	X	X
4	X	$\sqrt{}$
5	$\sqrt{}$	$\sqrt{}$
6	X	X
7	X	$\sqrt{}$
8	X	X
9	X	$\sqrt{}$
10	X	X
11	X	$\sqrt{}$
12	X	$\sqrt{}$
13	X	X
14	X	X
15	X	$\sqrt{}$
16	$\sqrt{}$	$\sqrt{}$
17	X	$\sqrt{}$
18	$\sqrt{}$	$\sqrt{}$
19	X	X
20	X	$\sqrt{}$

Physiotherapist	Opinions prior to receipt of factsheet	Opinions after the receipt of factsheet
21	X	X
22	X	√
23	X	X
24	√	√
25	X	X
26	X	X
27	√	X
28	X	√
29	X	√
30	X	√

State what your χ^2 value is and what your p value is. Write this out in a similar format to that given on page 108.

NON-PARAMETRIC STATISTICAL TEST FOR USE WITH SAME AND MATCHED SUBJECT DESIGNS, TWO CONDITIONS AND ORDINAL OR INTERVAL/RATIO DATA

Wilcoxon signed-ranks test

To recap, this test is used when you have two conditions (either one control condition and one experimental condition *or* two experimental conditions) and you have either *one* group of subjects doing both conditios, or two groups of *matched* subjects, one group doing one condition and the other group the other condition (see Designs 1a and 2a on pages 101–102). The data for this test *must be ordinal or interval/ratio*.

Essentially what the Wilcoxon test does is to compare the performance of each S (or pairs of matched Ss) in each condition to see if there is a significant difference between them. When you calculate this test, you end up with a numerical value for T which you then look up in the probability tables for the Wilcoxon test to see if this value represents a significant difference between the conditions.

Example

Let's take an example. The issue regarding the wearing of uniform by physiotherapists seems unresolved. Some physiotherapists are of the opinion that uniforms increase the psychological distance between the patient and therapist and thus discourage the development of rapport. Others feel that the nature of the physiotherapist's job can be very stressful and intimate; the uniform sanctions such activities and makes the patient feel more comfortable. Obviously central to this issue is the patient/therapist relationship — a factor of major importance in long-stay patients. You decide you will assess the effects of physiotherapists wearing uniform on the degree of confidence experienced by a group of long-stay patients. Therefore you decide to test the following hypothesis:

H_1 Long-stay patients experience greater confidence when being treated by uniformed physiotherapists than by non-uniformed physiotherapists.

(What would your null hypothesis be?)

You devise a questionnaire which simply asks the subject to indicate on a 5-point scale (ordinal data) how confident they feel when being treated (a) by a uniformed physiotherapist and (b) by a non-uniformed physiotherapist. On your scale, a score of 1 means 'not at all confident' while 5 means 'very confident'. You give this questionnaire to 15 paraplegic patients. Thus, you have the following design:

	Condition 1 Rating uniformed physios	Ratings are compared to see whether there is any significant
1 group of 15 paraplegic subjects *takes part in*		
takes part in	**Condition 2** Rating non-uniformed physios	difference in the degree of confidence experienced

You administer your questionnaire to the 15 Ss (having, of course, included all the essential pre-requisites for such a design — Chs 2 and 3) and you end up with the following results:

Results			**Calculations**			
Subject	1 Condition A Uniform	2 Condition B* Non-uniform	3 d = A − B	4 Rank of d	5 Rank of + differences	6 Rank of − differences
1	5	3	+ 2	(+) 5.5	+ 5.5	
2	4	3	+ 1	(+) 1.5	+ 1.5	
3	5	2	+ 3	(+) 9.5	+ 9.5	
4	2	5	− 3	(−) 9.5		− 9.5
5	4	4	0	exclude		
6	3	3	0	exclude		
7	5	4	+ 1	(+) 1.5	+ 1.5	
8	5	3	+ 2	(+) 5.5	+ 5.5	
9	4	2	+ 2	(+) 5.5	+ 5.5	
10	4	2	+ 2	(+) 5.5	+ 5.5	
11	2	2	0	exclude		
12	3	1	+ 2	(+) 5.5	+ 5.5	
13	5	1	+ 4	(+) 11.5	+ 11.5	
14	4	2	+ 2	(+) 5.5	+ 5.5	
15	5	1	+ 4	(+) 11.5	+ 11.5	
Σ	60	38			+ 68.5	− 9.5
$\bar{x}$	4	2.533				

* It does not matter which condition is called A and which B.

Calculating the Wilcoxon test

In order to find out whether these ratings differ significantly for each condition, you must take the following steps:

1. Add up the total (Σ) for the uniformed condition A
$$\Sigma A = 60$$
2. Add up the total (Σ) for the non-uniformed condition B
$$\Sigma B = 38$$
3. Find the mean ($\bar{x}$) for each condition
$$\bar{x}A = 4 \qquad \bar{x}B = 2.533$$
4. Calculate the difference(d) for each pair of scores by taking A − B, remembering to put in the + and −signs.
∴ for S1 you would have $5 - 3 = +2$ and so on. Put the results in column 3 (d = A − B).
5. You must then *rank order* these differences by giving a rank of 1 to the smallest difference, 2 to the next smallest and so on. When you do this, you must ignore the plus and minus signs. *However*, where the difference between a pair of scores is 0, you omit this pair *altogether* from the analysis. Therefore, in this example, subjects 5, 6 and 11 are now excluded from any further analysis.

   You will also note that there are a number of d values which are identical, e.g. Ss 2 and 7 both have a d of + 1, Ss 1, 8, 9, 10, 12 and 14 all have a d value of +2. Where this happens a special procedure is used — the *tied rank* procedure.

Tied rank procedure

To carry out the tied rank procedure, rank the scores as usual, giving a rank of 1 to the smallest, 2 to the next smallest (remember — we omit the Os and ignore the + and − values). Continue this procedure until you come to the tied scores. Here, Ss 2 and 7 *both* have d values of 1. What we do here, then, is to add up the ranks these two d values would have had, if they had been different (that is ranks 1 and 2) and divide this by the number of d values that are the same (i.e. 2 d values of 1).

$$\therefore \frac{1 + 2}{2} = 1.5$$

Therefore, the d values of 1 are both given the ranks of 1.5 (see column entitled Rank of d).

We now find there are 6 d values of 2. Had these values been different, they would have occupied ranks 3, 4, 5, 6, 7 and 8 (because ranks 1 and 2 have already been used up).
Therefore we add these ranks together:
$$3 + 4 + 5 + 6 + 7 + 8 = 33$$

and divide this by the number of d values which are the same (i.e. 6 d values of 2) = 33 ÷ 6 = 5.5.

Thus, all the d-values of 2 are assigned the rank 5.5

We now find there are 2 d values of 3 (Ss 3 and 4). Had these values been different, they would have occupied the ranks 9 and 10 (because ranks 1–8 have now been used up).

Therefore, we add these ranks together

9 + 10 = 19

and divide this by the number of d values which are the same (i.e. 2 d values of 3) which is 19 ÷ 2 = 9.5.

Therefore, both the d values of 3 are given the rank of 9.5.

Now there are only two remaining d values, each of which is 4. Had these d values been different they would have occupied ranks 11 and 12 (because ranks 1–10 have now been used up). Therefore we add these ranks together (11 + 12 = 23) and divide this by the number of d values which are the same (i.e. 2 d values of 4) = 11.5. Thus, the d values of 4 are each given the rank of 11.5

Many people get very irritated by this ranking procedure, especially when calculating tied ranks, because a slip of just one figure can throw everything out. To avoid this, you may wish to write out all the ranks you will be using and cross them off as you use them. Here, then, we would write out the following ranks

1, 2, 3, 4, 5, 6, 7, 8, 9, 10, 11, 12

and strike them off as we go along.

Remember, the highest rank should be the same as the number of differences between scores you are ranking. Here we are ranking 12 d values, so the highest rank will be 12.

6. Now write in by each rank the plus or minus sign of the corresponding d value. Therefore, the first rank of 5.5 is given a plus sign because it has a corresponding d value of + 2.

7. Put all the ranks with a + sign into column 5 'Rank of + differences'. Put all the ranks with a − sign into the column 6 'Rank of minus differences'.

8. Add up the ranks for the column 5 'Rank of + differences' to give the total (Σ) for the + ranks, i.e. + 68.5
Add up the ranks for the column 6 'Rank of − differences' to give the total (Σ) for the − ranks, i.e. − 9.5

9. Take the *smaller* of the two ranks, *ignoring* the plus or minus sign, as your value of T (i.e. T = 9.5).

10. Find N by counting up the number of subjects (or in the case of matched groups, *pairs* of Ss) omitting those who had d values of 0, i.e. 15 − 3 = 12.

Looking up the value of T for significance

To see whether this *T* value of 9.5 represents a significant difference in the confidence levels experienced with uniformed and non-uniformed physiotherapists, it must be looked up in the probability tables for the Wilcoxon test (Table A2.2).

Down the left-hand column you will see values of N, while across the top you will see Levels of Significance for one-and two-tailed tests. Under each of these are columns of figures which are called *critical values* of *T*.

To find out whether our *T* value is significant at one of the levels indicated, we must first locate our *N* value of 12 down the left-hand column. To the right of this you will see four numbers which represent the *critical values* of *T* for this number of Ss. These values are: 17   14   10   7. Each of these figures is associated with the corresponding p value indicated at the top of the column. For example, a critical value of 14 is associated with a probability of

0.05   for a two-tailed test

and 0.025 for a one-tailed test

In order for your *T* value to be significant at a given level, it has to be *equal to or smaller* than one of these four figures. So, taking our *T* value of 9.5, look at the first figure to the right of N = 12, i.e. 17. Our *T* value is *smaller* than 17, so look at the next figure — 14. Our *T* value is *smaller* than 14, so look at the next figure — 10. Our *T* value is *smaller* than 10, so look at the next figure — 7. Our *T* value is *larger* than 7.

Because we have a one-tailed hypothesis (*more* confidence with uniforms) this means our results are significant between the 0.01 and 0.005 (or 1%–½%) levels. Now, to be significant at a given level, the *T* value must be *equal* to or *smaller* than the critical value of *T*. Because it is smaller than 10 but larger than 7, we must select the value of 10, which is associated with a significance level of 1%. Had our *T* value equalled this figure exactly, we would say that our results are significant at *p equals* 0.01. However, our *T* value is smaller than 10,which means that its significance is actually less than 0.01. Therefore we express this as:

$p < 0.01$ (< means 'less than')

This means that the probability of our results being due to random error is less than 1%.

Interpreting the results

Our *T* value is associated with a *p* value of < 0.01 level (i.e. $< 1\%$ level) which means that there is less than a 1% chance that our results are due to random error. If you remember, we said a good rule of thumb for claiming support for your hypothesis is the 5% or 0.05 level. Because our *T* has a *smaller p* value than 5%, we can say that our results are significant. *But*, it is very important to note that you must check the averages for each set of data (A = 4, B = 2.533) to see whether the results are in the direction you predicted (i.e. larger on the uniform condition), since occasionally, you may get significant results which are actually the *reverse* of what you predicted and therefore would not support your hypothesis.

Here, the results *are* in the direction you predicted and therefore, we can say that your hypothesis has been supported (i.e. we can *reject* the *null* hypothesis).

We can state this in the following way:

Using a Wilcoxon test on the data ($T = 9.5$, $N = 12$), the results were found to be significant at $p < 0.01$ level for a one-tailed test. This suggests that long-stay patients experience greater degrees of confidence when being treated by a uniformed physiotherapist than by a non-uniformed physiotherapist.

[At what level would the results have been significant had the hypothesis been two-tailed?]

Activity 22 (Answers on pages 282–283)

1. To practise ranking, rank order the following results using the guidelines above. Remember to rank from smallest to biggest, omitting any zero scores, ignoring the plus and minus signs of the d values, and giving the average rank for tied d values.

Subject	Condition A	Condition B	d	Rank
1	10	9	+1	
2	8	9	−1	
3	9	7	+2	
4	6	7	−1	
5	5	4	+1	
6	8	3	+5	
7	7	6	+1	
8	9	9	0	
9	9	6	+3	
10	5	6	−1	
11	7	3	+4	
12	8	4	+4	

2. To practise looking up T values, look up the following and say whether you would classify them as significant
   - (i) $T = 7$ $N = 9$ one-tailed
   - (ii) $T = 7$ $N = 15$ two-tailed
   - (iii) $T = 15$ $N = 13$ one-tailed
   - (iv) $T = 20$ $N = 16$ one-tailed
   - (v) $T = 16$ $N = 12$ two-tailed
   - (vi) $T = 32$ $N = 16$ one-tailed
   - (vii) $T = 7$ $N = 12$ two-tailed
   - (viii) $T = 12$ $N = 13$ one-tailed

3. Calculate a Wilcoxon on the following data:

H_1 Traction is more effective than surgical collars for patients with cervical spondylosis.

Brief method. Select two groups of 12 cervical spondylosis patients, matched on sex, age, length and severity of condition, and previous treatments, and treat Group 1 with traction and Group 2 with surgical collars. After 3 weeks, compare the movement regained on a 7-point scale (1 = no improvement, 7 = greatly improved.)

Subject pair	Condition A Traction	Condition B Collar
1	3	3
2	4	3
3	5	4
4	4	3
5	7	3
6	4	4
7	4	4
8	6	5
9	5	3
10	3	2
11	6	3
12	4	3

Write down the T value
   N value
   p value
and state whether or not your results are significant, using the format of the paragraph on page 115.

NON-PARAMETRIC STATISTICAL TESTS FOR USE WITH SAME AND MATCHED SUBJECT DESIGNS, THREE OR MORE CONDITIONS AND ORDINAL OR INTERVAL/RATIO DATA

1. Friedman test

This test is similar to the Wilcoxon in that it is used for related and matched subject designs. However, the Friedman is used when either

a. *one* group of subjects is tested under *three or more* conditions; the results from the conditions are compared for differences.
   or
b. *three or more* groups of *matched* subjects are each tested in one condition; the results from the groups are compared for differences.

You would use this test if you had either Design 1b or 2b on page 102 and ordinal or interval/ratio data.

However, the Friedman test only tells you whether the results from each condition differ and not whether the results from one condition are better.

For this reason, any hypothesis which relates to the Friedman must predict general differences and not a specific direction to the results. In other words, it must be *two-tailed*. When calculating this test, you end up with a numerical value for χr^2 which you then look up in the probability tables associated with the Friedman test to see whether this represents a significant difference between your conditions.

Example

To illustrate this, let's suppose that you are a teacher in a large school of physiotherapy. You've noticed that over the last 2 or 3 years students seem to do consistently worse on the geriatric and neurology clinical placements, than on orthopaedic and cardiothoracic placements. This may be due to a number of factors, such as the quality of the theoretical preparation or clinical supervision. However, before moving on to find the cause, you must first establish whether or not your observation is correct. Your hypothesis is:

H_1 Third-year physiotherapy students perform differently in various clinical settings.

To test this hypothesis, you randomly select 17 students in the final year of their training and compare their marks (on a 10-point scale; 1 = disastrous, 10 = excellent) in four clinical settings — geriatric, neurology, orthopaedics and cardiothoracic.

Your design, then, looks like this:

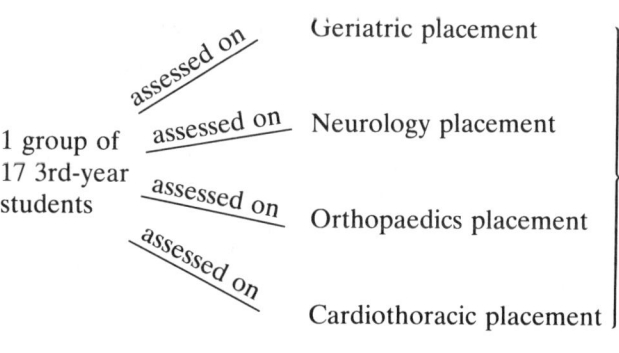

Your data is as follows:

Subject	Condition A Geriatric Score	Rank	Condition B Neurology Score	Rank	Condition C Orthopaedics Score	Rank	Condition D Cardiothoracic Score	Rank
1	5	1	6	2	8	4	7	3
2	6	2.5	6	2.5	7	4	5	1
3	3	1	7	3.5	7	3.5	6	2
4	8	2	9	3	10	4	7	1
5	7	1.5	9	3.5	9	3.5	7	1.5
6	6	1.5	8	3	9	4	6	1.5
7	5	1	8	3	9	4	7	2
8	5	1	8	2.5	10	4	8	2.5
9	4	1	6	2	8	3	9	4
10	3	1	5	2	8	4	7	3
11	6	2	5	1	8	4	7	3
12	6	2.5	4	1	7	4	6	2.5
13	7	2	5	1	9	4	8	3
14	3	1	7	3	8	4	6	2
15	2	1	5	2	7	3.5	7	3.5
16	5	1	6	2.5	7	4	6	2.5
17	4	1	6	2	7	3.5	7	3.5
	$\Sigma = 85$	$T_c = 24$	$\Sigma = 110$	$T_c = 39.5$	$\Sigma = 138$	$T_c = 65$	$\Sigma = 116$	$T_c = 41.5$
	$\bar{x} = 5$		$\bar{x} = 6.471$		$\bar{x} = 8.118$		$\bar{x} = 6.824$	

Calculating the Friedman test

In order to calculate the Friedman you must take the following steps:
1. Firstly, add up the scores for each condition
   $$\therefore \Sigma A = 85 \quad \Sigma B = 110 \quad \Sigma C = 138 \quad \Sigma D = 116$$
2. Find out the means for each condition
   $$\therefore \bar{x}A = 5 \quad \bar{x}B = 6.471 \quad \bar{x}C = 8.118 \quad \bar{x}D = 6.824$$
3. Rank the scores for each subject (i.e. *across* the row) giving the rank of 1 to the smallest score, a rank of 2 to the next smallest and so on. You will only need ranks 1–4 as there are only four scores for each subject. Where you have tied scores, use the tied rank procedure (see pp 112–113) i.e. add up the ranks these scores would have had if they had been different, and divide by the number of scores which are the same. Therefore, if we look at subject 2, she scored 5 in cardiothoracic, 6 in geriatric, 6 in neurology and 7 in orthopaedics. Thus 5 gets a rank of 1; the two 6s, had they been different would have had ranks of 2 and 3 (because rank 1 has now been used up); so we add 2 and 3 = 5, and divide this by the total number of scores which are the same (i.e. 2, because there are 2 6s) = 2.5. This, then is the rank we give the 6s. The score of 7 in orthopaedics gets a rank of 4 because ranks 1–3 have been used up.
4. Now add up the ranks for each condition (i.e. for each clinical setting). This is called T_c
   $$T_c \text{ for A} = 24 \quad T_c \text{ for B} = 39.5$$
   $$T_c \text{ for C} = 65 \quad T_c \text{ for D} = 41.5$$

5. You now have to find the value of χr^2 from the following formula:

$$\chi r^2 = \left[\left(\frac{12}{NC\,(C+1)}\right)(\Sigma T_c^2)\right] - 3\,N\,(C+1)$$

where N = number of Ss in the group (or in the case of matched designs, the number of sets of subjects)
i.e. 17

C = number of conditions
i.e. 4

T_c = total of the ranks for each condition
T_c for condition A = 24
T_c for condition B = 39.5
T_c for condition C = 65
T_c for condition D = 41.5

T_c^2 = each rank total squared
i.e. 24^2; 39.5^2; 65^2; 41.5^2
= 576; 1560.25; 4225; 1722.25

Σ = sum or total of all the calculations following it

ΣT_c^2 = the sum of the squared ranks for each condition
i.e. 576 + 1560.25 + 4225 + 1722.25
= 8083.5

Remember! Do all the calculations in brackets first, starting with divisions and multiplications and finally additions and subtractions.

Thus, if we substitute some values in the formula:

$$\chi r^2 = \left[\left(\frac{12}{17 \times 4\,(4+1)}\right) \times (576 + 1560.25 + 4225 + 1722.25)\right]$$
$$- 3 \times 17\,(4+1)$$

$$= \left[\left(\frac{12}{68 \times 5}\right) \times (567 + 1560.25 + 4225 + 1722.25)\right] - 51 \times 5$$

$$= [0.035 \times 8083.5] - 255$$
$$= 282.923 - 255$$
$$\therefore \chi r^2 = 27.923$$

Looking up the value of χr^2

To look up χr^2 in the tables, you also need the degrees of freedom value — this is the number of conditions minus 1, i.e. $4 - 1 = 3$. As you will see, there are three main tables for the Friedman test — Tables A2.3a, 3b and 1. Table A2.3a is used where there are three conditions and only 2–9 subjects in each condition; Table A2.3b is for four conditions, with 2–4 Ss in each, and Table A2.1 is for anything larger, i.e. more conditions or more subjects.

Because we have four conditions and 17 subjects, we must use Table A2.1. (This table is also for use with the χ^2 test.) You will see that in the left-hand column, entitled df, there are various degrees of freedom values. Look down this column until you have found the df for this example, i.e. 3. You will see five numbers called *critical values* to the right — 6.25, 7.82, 9.84, 11.34 and 16.27. Each of these values is associated with the level of probability shown at the top of its column, e.g. 11.34 is associated with a *p* value of 0.01. To be significant at a given level, our χr^2 value must be *equal* to or *larger* than the values here. So, if we take the first value 6.25, our χr^2 value is larger; it is also larger than 7.82, 9.84, 11.34 and 16.27. Therefore we take the value 16.27 and look up the column to see what the associated level of significance is, i.e. 0.001 or the 0.1% level. Because our χr^2 value of 27.923 is *larger* than the critical value of 16.27, this means that our results are significant at *less than* ($<$) the 0.001 level. (Had our χr^2 value been 16.27 *exactly*, we would say our *p* value *equals* 0.001.)

This means that there is less than a 0.1% chance that our results are due to random error.

Note that because the Friedman *only* allows you to predict differences and *not* specific directions to the results, your hypothesis must be two-tailed and so this level of significance represents the level for a two-tailed hypothesis. Because our usual cut-off point is 5% and our *p* value is less than that, i.e. 0.1%, we can say that our results are significant at $< 0.1\%$ level.

Interpreting the results

The results are associated with a *p* value of less than 0.1%. This means that there is less than a 0.1% probability of our results being due to random error. As the standard cut-off point is 5%, we can reject our null hypothesis and say that our results are significant. In other words, students do perform differently in a variety of clinical settings. We can express this in the following way:

> Using a Friedman test on the data ($\chi r^2 = 27.923$, $N = 17$), the results were found to be significant at $p < 0.001$, for a two-tailed test. This suggests that 3rd-year physiotherapy students perform significantly differently in four clinical settings, and so supports the experimental hypothesis. The null hypothesis can therefore be rejected.

Do note, however, that the Friedman only allows us to identify differences and not to say in which setting they performed better. If, however, you do expect a trend in the results of a related or matched subject design (e.g. that students do worst in geriatrics, followed by cardiothoracic, followed by neurology and best in orthopaedics, you would need the Page's *L* trend test — see next section).

If you had only three conditions and fewer subjects then you would use Table A2.3a. For example, supposing you had three conditions and seven subjects, and a χr^2 value of 7.5 you would look to find your value of N across the top of the table, (remember N = the number of Ss or subject pairs). Under this you will see a column for the χr^2 value, and to the right the corresponding p value or significance level. So taking the column for N = 7, look down the χr^2 value to find 7.5. Since our χr^2 value must be *equal* to or *larger* than those given to be significant at a given level, we find that our value of 7.5 is larger than 7.143, but smaller than 7.714. We must take the critical value of 7.143 (because our χr^2 value must be *equal to* or *larger* than the critical value given) which gives us a corresponding p value of 0.027 or 2.7%.

However, because our χr^2 value of 7.5 is larger than 7.143, this means our p value is even *less than* (<) 0.027. Had our χr^2 value equalled the critical value of 7.143, we would say that our p value *equals* 0.027. So, our results have a p value of < 0.027. Using the standard cut-off of 0.05, we can say our results are significant. We can therefore *reject* the *null* hypothesis, and *accept* the *experimental* hypothesis.

Supposing, however, we had four conditions, and four subjects or pairs of subjects and a χr^2 value of 2.6, we would need to use Table A2.3b which is for use with four conditions and 2–4 Ss. Here we would find the column corresponding to our N value, and look down the χr^2 values to find our own of 2.6. Because our value has to be equal to or larger than the values given to be significant at a given level, we can see that our χr^2 value of 2.6 is larger than 2.4 but smaller than 2.7. Therefore we have to take the value next smallest to our own, i.e. 2.4, which gives us a p value of 0.524 or 52.4%. Because of our standard 5% cut-off point, this p value cannot be classified as significant because it is larger. Therefore we would have to conclude that our results were not significant, our hypothesis was not supported and we would have to accept the null (no relationship) hypothesis.

Activity 23 (Answers on page 283)

1. To practise looking up χr^2 values, look up the following and say whether they are significant
   - (i) $C = 4$ $N = 3$ $\chi r^2 = 7.4$ p
   - (ii) $C = 4$ $N = 10$ $\chi r^2 = 9.92$ p
   - (iii) $C = 3$ $N = 6$ $\chi r^2 = 5.72$ p
   - (iv) $C = 3$ $N = 12$ $\chi r^2 = 35.7$ p
   - (v) $C = 3$ $N = 8$ $\chi r^2 = 9.3$ p
2. Calculate a Friedman on the following data:

   H_1 The muscle tone of the quadriceps in children differs for Asians, Caucasians and West Indians.

   Method   Select seven children in each racial group, matched for age, sex, fitness, activity levels and compare their muscle tone, using a 5-point scale: 5 = very high tone and 1 = very poor tone.

S	Condition A Asian	Condition B Caucasian	Condition C West Indian
1	3	4	5
2	2	2	5
3	2	3	4
4	1	2	3
5	3	2	2
6	1	2	1
7	3	3	3

Write down the χr^2 value and the p value. State whether or not your results are significant, and what they mean, using the example given on page 120.

2. Page's L trend test

This test is an extension of the Friedman test, in that it is used when
  a. the design is a related or matched subject one
  b. the data is ordinal or interval/ratio
  c. there are three or more conditions (i.e. one group of Ss doing three or more conditions, or three or more *matched* groups of Ss each doing one condition).

However, there is one salient difference — whereas the Friedman test can only be used to discover whether there are *differences* between the conditions without saying which condition is significantly better or worse than the others, the Page's L trend test is used when the experimenter had predicted a *trend* in the results; for example when comparing the quality of three schools of physiotherapy, the experimenter, *in the hypothesis*, predicts that School A is better than School B, which in turn is better than School C. This contrasts with the sort of hypothesis which must be used with the Friedman test, which would simply predict *differences* in quality between the three schools. Thus the sort of design we might have with the Page's L trend test is:

1. In a comparison of a group of students' attitudes to three types of teaching method, it is predicted that the seminar method will be most popular, followed by the lecture method with tutorials least popular

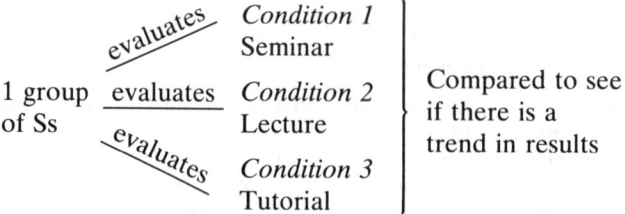

or alternatively, the following design is appropriate for use with the Page's L trend test:

2. In a comparison of three types of exercise techniques following prostatectomy, it is predicted that Exercise A will be more effective than
Exercise B which will be more effective than Exercise C. Three groups
of patients, matched for age, duration of illness, length of time post-op,
severity of illness etc, are given one of the exercise regimes and compared
for continence after 1 month.

matched on certain key variables {

Group 1	uses	Exercise A	Compared for
Group 2	uses	Exercise B	a trend in the
Group 3	uses	Exercise C	results

The Page's L trend test then essentially assesses whether there is a significant trend in the results. When calculating it you derive the value of L,
which is then looked up in the probability tables associated with the Page's
test to see whether this value represents a significant trend in your results.

Because you are predicting a specific direction to the results when you
use a Page's L trend test, the hypothesis must be one-tailed.

Example

Let's take the first hypothesis that in order to evaluate students' preferences
for three types of teaching approach, you predict that the seminar method
will be more popular than the lecture method, with the tutorial being least
popular — a *trend* is predicted, i.e. seminar > lecture > tutorial (> means
'greater than').

You select a group of 10 students and ask them to rate the three methods
on a 5-point scale (5 = most preferred, 1 = least preferred). In order to
analyse the results you *must* set out your data such that the scores you
predict will be the *smallest* (i.e. tutorial) are placed on the left, and the
scores you predict to be the *largest* are placed on the *right* thus:

Subject	Condition 1 Tutorial		Condition 2 Lecture		Condition 3 Seminar	
	Score	Rank	Score	Rank	Score	Rank
1	3	1.5	4	3	3	1.5
2	2	1.5	2	1.5	4	3
3	3	1.5	3	1.5	5	3
4	1	1	3	3	2	2
5	2	1.5	3	3	2	1.5
6	2	1	4	2	5	3
7	1	1	2	2	4	3
8	3	1	4	2.5	4	2.5
9	2	1	4	2	5	3
10	1	1	3	2	4	3
	$\Sigma_1 = 20$	$T_c 1 = 12$	$\Sigma_2 = 32$	$T_c{}^2 = 22.5$	$\Sigma_3 = 38$	$T_c{}^3 = 25.5$

Calculating the Page's L trend test

1. In order to calculate the value of L you must take the following steps:
First find the total scores for each condition
$\Sigma_1 = 20$ $\Sigma_2 = 32$ $\Sigma_3 = 38$
Then find the mean score for each condition
$\bar{x}_1 = 2$ $\bar{x}_2 = 3.2$ $x_3 = 3.8$
2. Rank the scores for each subject (or sets of *matched* Ss) across the row, as for the Friedman, giving the rank of 1 to the lowest score, the rank of 2 to the next lowest etc. If you have two or more scores which are the same, you must give these the *average* rank (see pages 112–113 on how to deal with tied scores), i.e. you add up the value of the ranks they would have obtained had they been different and divide by the number of scores that are the same. Therefore, S1 has two scores of 3. Had these scores been different they would have had the ranks 1 and 2. These values are added together (3) and divided by 2 (because there are *two* scores of 3) to give the average rank, 1.5, which is entered alongside the scores of 3.
3. Add up the ranks for each condition
i.e. $T_c1 = 12$ $T_c2 = 22.5$ $T_c3 = 25.5$
4. Find the value of L from the formula
$$L = \Sigma(T_c1 \times c) + \Sigma(T_c2 \times c) + \Sigma(T_c3 \times c)$$
Where: Σ means the total or sum of any symbols that follow it
T_c = total of ranks for each condition
i.e. $T_c1 = 12$; $T_c2 = 22.5$; $T_c3 = 25.5$
c = numbers allotted to the conditions from left to right
i.e. 1, 2 and 3
$(T_c \times c)$ = total of the ranks for each condition multiplied by the number assigned to the condition
i.e. $T_c1 \times 1 = 12 \times 1$
$T_c2 \times 2 = 22.5 \times 2$
$T_c3 \times 3 = 25.5 \times 3$
$L = (12 \times 1) + (22.5 \times 2) + (25.5 \times 3)$
$= 12 + 45 + 76.5$
$= 133.5$
5. To look up your value of L, you also need two further values — C (the number of conditions, i.e. 3) and N (the number of Ss in the group or the number of sets of matched Ss, i.e. 10).

Looking up the value of L for significance

Turn to Table A2.4. Across the top you will see values of C (i.e. number of conditions) from 3 to 6, and down the left-hand column, values of N (i.e. number of Ss or sets of matched Ss) from 2 to 12. Look across the c values to find our value of $C = 3$ and down the N values to find our $N = 10$ value.

At their intersection point you will see three numbers — 134, 131, and 128. These are called *critical values* of L. If you look across these rows to the right-hand column, you will see that 134 represents a p value of 0.001; 131 represents a p value of 0.01 and 128 represents a p value of 0.05. To be significant at one of these levels, your L value must be *equal* to or *larger* than one of the numbers 134, 131 and 128. The obtained value of L in our example is 133.5. This is larger than 131, but smaller than 134. Therefore we must take the value of 131, which represents a significance level of 0.01 or 1%. But because our L value is *larger* than the critical value of 131, this means that the corresponding p value is *less than* (<) 0.01. This is expressed as $p < 0.01$. This means that there is less than a 1% chance of the results being caused by random error. Because you *must* be predicting a specific direction to your results in order to be using a trend test, your hypothesis, by definition, must be one-tailed. Therefore, all the values in this table are values for a one-tailed hypothesis.

Using our usual cut-off point of 5%, because the p value in our study is smaller, we can conclude that our results are significant at < 0.01 level. Thus we can reject the null hypothesis and conclude that there is a significant trend in results as predicted in our hypothesis.

Interpreting the results

Our results have a probability value of < 0.01 which means that there is less than a 1% chance of them being due to random error. Because this p value is *smaller* than the usual cut-off point of 0.05, we can say that our results are significant. This means we can *reject* the null hypothesis and *accept* the *experimental* hypothesis.

This can be expressed in the following way:

Using a Page's L trend test on the data ($L = 133.5$, $N = 10$, $C = 3$), the results were found to be significant at $p < 0.01$ for a one-tailed hypothesis. This suggests that the experimental hypothesis has been supported, and that students prefer seminar teaching methods to lectures, with tutorials being the least preferred approach. The null hypothesis can therefore be rejected.

Activity 24 (Answers on page 283)

1. To practise looking up L values, look up the following and decide at what level (if any) they are significant:
   (i) $N = 5$ $C = 4$ $L = 142.5$ p
   (ii) $N = 8$ $C = 5$ $L = 384$ p
   (iii) $N = 7$ $C = 3$ $L = 92$ p
   (iv) $N = 12$ $C = 6$ $L = 971$ p
   (v) $N = 10$ $C = 5$ $L = 455.5$ p
2. Calculate a Page's L trend test on the following data:
        H_1 It is hypothesised that hydrotherapy is more effective than exercise

which in turn is more effective than massage for mobilising lower limbs paralysed following a stroke.

Method Take three groups, each of 8 subbjects, matched for severity of paralysis, age, sex, previous health, length of time since stroke and other treatments, and give each group one of the three treatment procedures. After 1 month compare the percentage range of movement regained. The results are as follows:

Subject trio	Condition 1 Hydrotherapy Score	Rank	Condition 2 Massage Score	Rank	Condition 3 Exercise Score	Rank
1	40		25		30	
2	55		30		40	
3	35		35		45	
4	20		30		40	
5	30		20		30	
6	50		45		50	
7	55		45		55	
8	60		50		60	

State your L and p values, using the sample format given on page 125.

Remember! Put the scores which are predicted to be the lowest in the left-hand column and those predicted to be the highest in the right-hand column.

Remember, too, that the data in this example is of an interval/ratio type, which can be used with both non-parametric and parametric tests.

8

Parametric tests for same and matched subject designs

All the statistical tests described in this chapter, like those in the previous one, are used to analyse the results from same subject or matched subject designs — in other words, those designs which either use *one* group of subjects for *all* the conditions, or alternatively, two or more groups of *matched* subjects who do one condition each (see pp. 91–93 for the designs).

There is one major difference, however; all the tests in this chapter are *parametric*, which means that they require certain conditions to be fulfilled before they can be used — in particular that the data must be of an interval/ratio level. They are also rather more difficult to calculate than non-parametric tests. You should always remember that for any given design, the relevant parametric and non-parametric tests do exactly the same job — they assess whether there are significant differences (or in the case of correlations, similarities) between the conditions, but the parametric tests are just more sensitive to these differences.

The designs we are interested in then are as follows:

1. One group of subjects used in all the conditions (same subject design)

a. Two conditions only

1 group of subjects — takes part in → *Condition 1*
— takes part in → *Condition 2*

Results from conditions compared for differences

b. Three or more conditions

1 group of subjects — takes part in → *Condition 1*
— takes part in → *Condition 2*
— takes part in → *Condition 3* (etc.)

Results from conditions compared for differences

2. Two or more groups of matched subjects, each of which is used in one condition only (matched subject designs)

a. Two matched groups only

matched on certain key variables
{

| Subject group 1 | takes part in | *Condition 1* | Results from conditions compared for differences |
| Subject group 2 | takes part in | *Condition 2* | |

b. Three or more matched groups

matched on certain key variables
{

Subject group 1	takes part in	*Condition 1*	Results from conditions compared for differences
Subject group 2	takes part in	*Condition 2*	
Subject group 3 (etc.)	takes part in	*Condition 3*	

Results from designs which use *one* group of subjects in both of *two* conditions (Design 1a) or *two* groups of matched subjects, doing *one* condition each (Design 2a) are analysed using the *related t-test*. Results from designs using *one* group of subjects in *three or more* conditions (Design 1b) or *three or more* groups of matched subjects doing one condition each (Design 2b) are analysed during the one-way analysis of variance (or anova as it is usually known) for related designs. In addition we shall look at the Scheffé multiple range test which is used in conjunction with the anova — see the relevant section.

Table 8.1 Parametric tests for related and matched subject designs

Design	Parametric test
1. One group of Ss tested under two conditions	Related *t* test
2. Two groups of *matched* Ss, each tested in one condition only	Related *t* test
3. One group of Ss tested under three or more conditions	One-way anova for related designs, to be used with the Scheffé multiple range test
4. Three or more groups of *matched* Ss, each tested in one condition only	One-way anova for related designs, to be used with the Scheffé multiple range test

PARAMETRIC STATISTICAL TEST FOR USE WITH ONE GROUP OF SUBJECTS AND TWO CONDITIONS OR TWO GROUPS OF MATCHED SUBJECTS, DOING ONE CONDITION EACH

Related t test

Just to recap, this test is used for exactly the same designs as the Wilcoxon, in other words, *one* group of subjects who take part in *two* conditions (a same subjects design) and the results from the two conditions are then compared for differences. Alternatively, the related t test is used where you have *two* groups of matched subjects, who do one condition each (a matched subject design) and again the results from the two conditions are compared to see if there are differences between them.

The related *t* test is especially suitable for 'before and after' type designs, for instance, when you wish to compare the effects of a treatment on one group of subjects.

When calculating the *t* test, you find the value of *t*, which you then look up in the probability tables for the *t* test to see whether this value represents significant differences between the results from each condition. Remember that parametric tests are more difficult to calculate than non-parametric tests, so don't panic when you look at the formula. As long as you work through the stages systematically, you will have no difficulty.

Example

Let's suppose you are in charge of a large physiotherapy department and it has been brought to your notice that the eight basic grade physiotherapists seem to show a distinct preference for treating young male sports injury leg fracture patients as opposed to elderly male leg fracture patients. You have challenged them about this but they deny it, so you want to produce some empirical support for your assertion.

Your experimental hypothesis, then, is:

H_1 That young male leg fracture patients receive more attention from basic grade physiotherapists than do elderly leg fracture patients.

To test your hypothesis, you measure the length of time each physiotherapist spends with her three sports injury fracture patients in the course of 1 day and total this up in minutes. You do the same for the period spent with her three elderly leg fracture patients. Because time is an Interval/Ratio measurement the most necessary condition for using a parametric test can be fulfilled.

Therefore you have the following design:

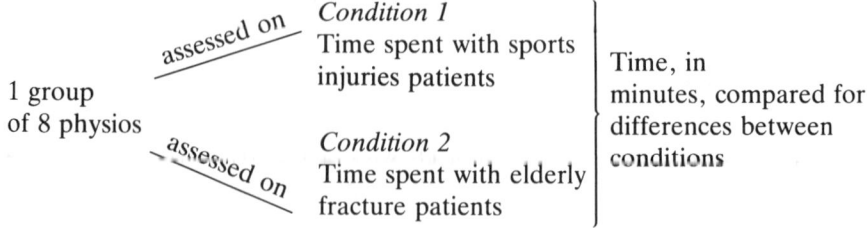

1 group of 8 physios | Condition 1 Time spent with sports injuries patients / Condition 2 Time spent with elderly fracture patients | Time, in minutes, compared for differences between conditions

Your results are as follows:

Results from Experiment			Calculations from statistical test	
1 Subject	2 *Condition 1* Sports injury	3 *Condition 2* Elderly patients	4 *d* (A − B)	5 *d²*
1	49	42	+ 7	49
2	57	45	+ 12	144
3	72	65	+ 7	49
4	64	65	− 1	1
5	50	60	− 10	100
6	45	35	+ 10	100
7	59	40	+ 19	361
8	65	49	+ 16	256
Σ	461	401	$\Sigma d = 60$	$\Sigma d^2 = 1060$
$\bar{x}$	57.625	50.125		

* It does not matter which group of patients is called Condition A and which Condition B.

Calculating the related t test

To calculate the related *t* test, you must first:
1. Add up the scores for each condition to give the total (Σ), i.e. $\Sigma A = 461$; $\Sigma B = 401$.
2. Calculate the mean score ($\bar{x}$) for each condition, i.e. $\bar{x}A = 57.625$; $\bar{x}B = 50.125$
3. Calculate the difference between each subject's pair of scores·and enter this in column 4(d), i.e. for each subject take the score of Condition B away from the score of Condition A (e.g. for S1, 49 − 42 = 7). Remember to put in the plus and minus signs, for each d value.
4. Add these differences up to give Σd, remembering to take account of the plus and minus values, i.e. $\Sigma d = 60$.
5. Square each difference to give d^2, i.e. $7^2 = 49$ and enter these in Column 5 (d^2).
6. Add up the d^2 values to give Σd^2, i.e. $\Sigma d^2 = 1060$.
7. Square the total of the differences, i.e. $60^2 = 3600$ to give $(\Sigma d)^2$. It is important to recognise the difference in meaning between

Σd^2 (Stage 6) which means to add up all the squared differences and
$(\Sigma d)^2$ (Stage 7) which means to add up all the differences and square the total.

8. Find the t from the following formula:

$$t = \frac{\Sigma d}{\sqrt{\dfrac{N \Sigma d^2 - (\Sigma d)^2}{N - 1}}}$$

where Σd = the total of the differences (i.e. 60)
$(\Sigma d)^2$ = the total of the differences, squared (i.e. 3600)
Σd^2 = the total of the squared differences (i.e. 1060)
N = number of subjects, or pairs of matched subjects (i.e. 8)
$\sqrt{}$ = the square root of the final calculation of everything under the square root sign.

If we substitute some values, then:

$$t = \frac{60}{\sqrt{\dfrac{8 \times 1060 - 3600}{8 - 1}}}$$

$$= \frac{60}{\sqrt{\dfrac{8480 - 3600}{7}}}$$

$$= \frac{60}{\sqrt{697.143}}$$

$$= \frac{60}{26.404}$$

$$t = 2.272$$

Looking up the value of t

To see whether this t value is significant you need one further value — the degrees of freedom — which here is the number of subjects minus 1, i.e. $8 - 1 = 7$. Turn to Table A2.5. You will see down the left-hand margin a number of df values. Look down the column until you find the df value of 7. To the right of that you will see 6 *critical values* of t:

1.415   1.895   2.365   2.998   3.499   5.405

If your value of t is *equal* to or *larger* than any of the given values, it is significant at the level indicated at the top of the column. For example, 3.499 has an associated p value of 0.005 for a one-tailed test and 0.01 for a two-tailed test. So, if we look at the numbers, we can see that our t value of

2.272 is larger than 1.895 but smaller than 2.365. We must select the critical value of 1.895, since to be significant at a given level our t value must be *equal to* or *larger than* the given value in the table. At the top of this column you will see a level of significance for both one- and two-tailed hypotheses. As we predicted that basic grades would spend *more* time with sports injury patients, we have a one-tailed hypothesis. This means that the probability that our results are due to random error is

less than 0.05, since our t value is *larger* than 1.895

We express this as: $p < 0.05$ ($<$ means 'less than')
(Had our t value been exactly the same as the critical value of 1.895 in the table, we would have said that $p = 0.05$.)

Interpreting the results

Our results have an associated probability of less than 0.05, which means that the chances of random error accounting for the outcome of our experiment are less than 5 in 100. Because the usual cut-off point for claiming that the results are significant is 5%, we can conclude that our results are significant, at less than 5% level. However, we can only say that our hypothesis has been supported if the results are in the direction predicted. This means that providing the average amount of time spent with the sports injury patients is greater than the average amount of time spent with the elderly leg fracture patients, we can reject the null hypothesis and accept that our experimental hypothesis has been supported. Since the averages are 57.625 and 50.125 minutes respectively, the results are in the predicted direction and we can conclude that basic grade physiotherapists spend significantly more time with young sports injury patients than elderly leg fracture patients. We can state this as follows:

Using a related t test on the data ($t = 2.272$, $N = 8$), the results are significant at $p < 0.05$, for a one-tailed test. The experimental hypothesis has been supported, suggesting that young male fracture patients receive significantly more treatment time from basic grade physiotherapists, than do elderly male fracture patients. The null hypothesis can therefore be rejected.

Remember, had the average time been reversed (i.e. more time spent with the elderly patients) we could *not* claim that the hypothesis had been supported.

Activity 25 (Answers on page 284)

1. To practise looking up t values, look up the following and say whether or not they are significant and at what level.
   (i) df = 11 $t = 2.406$ one-tailed p
   (ii) df = 14 $t = 1.895$ two-tailed p
   (iii) df = 19 $t = 2.739$ one-tailed p

(iv) df = 7 $t = 3.204$ one-tailed p
(v) df = 9 $t = 2.973$ two-tailed p

2. Calculate a related t test on the following data:

> H_1 Student physiotherapists with 'A'-level physics do better on their 1st year theory exam than students without 'A'-level physics.
>
> Method Select two groups, each of 12 students, matched on certain key features such as overall 'A'-level points, attendance levels, quality of teaching etc. Of these, one group has 'A'-level physics and the other does not. Compare the performance of the two groups on their 1st year theory exam. The marks are as follows.

Results from experiment			Calculations from statistical test	
1	2	3	4	5
Subject pair	*Condition 1* 'A'-level physics	*Condition 2* No 'A' level physics	d	d^2
1	64	68		
2	59	60		
3	72	62		
4	68	58		
5	58	49		
6	70	62		
7	65	61		
8	62	50		
9	73	71		
10	45	49		
11	56	54		
12	67	68		

State the t value, the df value, and the p value expressed in a similar format to that on page 132.

PARAMETRIC STATISTICAL TESTS FOR USE WITH ONE GROUP OF SUBJECTS AND THREE OR MORE CONDITIONS OR THREE OR MORE GROUPS OF MATCHED SUBJECTS

One-way analysis of variance (anova) for related and matched subject designs

The one-way anova for related and matched subject designs is the parametric equivalent of the Friedman test. In other words it is used for designs which *either* use one subject group in three or more conditions and the results from these conditions are compared for differences between them. Or alternatively, it is used where the experimenter has got three or more groups of matched subjects who do one condition each. The results from each condition are compared for differences (see Designs 1b and 2b pp 127–128).

It is called a *one-way* anova because it only deals with experiments which manipulate *one* independent variable. If you ever hypothesised a relationship between *two* independent variables and a DV (see Ch. 3) you would require a two-way anova, or in extremis a relationship between *three* independent variables and a DV, then you would require a three-way anova. However, these are outside the scope of this book and the reader is referred to Greene & D'Oliveira (1982) and Ferguson (1976).

Like all parametric tests, the data must be of an interval/ratio level, and the remaining three conditions should be more or less fulfilled.

When calculating an anova you find the value of F which is then looked up in the probability tables for anovas to find out whether this value represents a significant difference between conditions. Like the Friedman test, the anova only tells us whether there are overall differences between conditions, and not the direction of the differences and so the hypothesis must be two-tailed.

Example

Because the anova is quite complicated to calculate, it may be helpful to explain the purpose of it beforehand. Let's imagine that you have noticed that your senior II physiotherapists seem to show a high degree of clinical skill but they seem less competent in their supervision of trainees and in their interpersonal skills. Obviously, if your observations are correct, you will need to do some staff development on the weaker areas. You therefore decide to make an evaluation of a group of 10 senior II physios in the three different aspects of their job — clinical skills, interpersonal skills and supervision skills.

Your hypothesis then is

H_1 Senior II physiotherapists show different levels of professional competence in three aspects of their job — clinical, supervisory and interpersonal skills.

To see if there is any difference in the competence shown in these areas you decide to compare the performance of the group on each aspect, giving marks out of 20. As this is an interval/ratio scale of measurement, we can fulfil this requirement of a parametric test.

Therefore we have the following design:

	assessed on clinical skills	
1 group of 10 senior IIs	assessed on interpersonal skills	Compared for differences in competence
	assessed on supervision skills	

Further suppose that you have collected and set out the results which look like this:

Subject	Condition 1 Clinical	Condition 2 Interpersonal	Condition 3 Supervisory	Total for Ss: T_s
1	15	12	11	38
2	12	9	8	29
3	13	10	11	34
4	10	10	12	32
5	17	14	10	41
6	8	12	11	31
7	11	12	9	32
8	14	9	9	32
9	16	8	12	36
10	10	9	8	27
Total T_c	$T_c1 = 126$	$T_c2 = 105$	$T_c3 = 101$	Grand total = 332

You are hypothesising that the performance of the group varies according to the aspect of the job, and therefore you would expect there to be significant differences or *variations* between the condition totals (126, 105 and 101). This, obviously, is one potential source of variation in the results and is called a *between-conditions* comparison. However, because each subject is assessed on all three conditions, we can also compare the overall performances of the subjects, to see if there is any variation in competence *between the physiotherapists*, i.e. a comparison of the total T_s totals. This comparison allows us to look at another potential source of variation in the scores — a *between-the-subjects* comparison. This is illustrated below for the example given above using the data from the first 5 subjects:

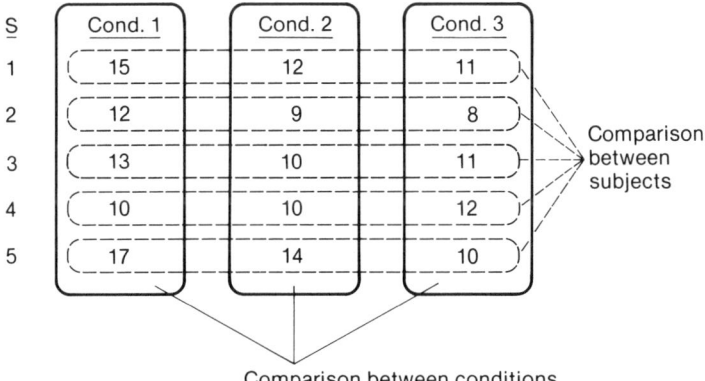

Comparison between conditions

Fig. 31

The solid vertical lines indicate the comparisons which can be made between conditions, to see if there is any difference in performance on each aspect of the job, as was hypothesised. This comparison concentrates on one source of potential variation in the results — the between-conditions variation. The dotted horizontal lines indicate the comparisons which can be made between subjects, to see if there is any difference in the *overall* performances among the *subjects*. This comparison concentrates on a second potential source of variation in the results — the between-subject variation. There is, of course, a third source of potential variation in scores — that due to *random error*.

If we consider these sources of variation for a moment, it can be seen that *ideally* what we would hope to find from our anova is:

a. significant differences between the performance of the job tasks, i.e. a significant *between-conditions* comparison, since this was what was hypothesised.

b. no significant differences between the subjects, since this would mean that they were not an atypical sample.

The purpose of the one-way related anova is to find out whether any of these sources of variation are responsible for significant differences in results.

In order to do this, we need a number of values:

the sums of squares	(SS)
the degrees of freedom	(df)
the mean squares	(MS)
the F ratios	(F)

for each source of variation. When these have been calculated they are entered into a table shown in the following format.

Source of variation of scores	Sums of squares (SS)	Degrees of freedom (df)	Mean squares (MS)	F ratios (F)
Variation *between conditions*, i.e. aspects of job	SS_{bet}	df_{bet}	MS_{bet}	F_{bet}
Variation between *subjects'* overall performance	SS_{subj}	df_{subj}	MS_{subj}	F_{subj}
Variation due to random *error*	SS_{error}	df_{error}	MS_{error}	
Total	SS_{tot}	df_{tot}		

Firstly, do not panic — the calculations are surprisingly easy, if rather laborious! Follow the steps described below (the data are on page 135).

Calculating the one-way anova

1. We must first calculate the SS values for each source of variation. To do this, you will need several values:

ΣT_c^2 = sum of the squared totals for each condition
i.e. $126^2 + 105^2 + 101^2$
= $15876 + 11025 + 10201$
= 37102

ΣT_s^2 = sum of each subject's performance squared
i.e. $38^2 + 29^2 + 34^2 + 32^2 + 41^2 + 31^2$
$+ 32^2 + 32^2 + 36^2 + 27^2$
= $1444 + 841 + 1156 + 1024 + 1681 +$
$961 + 1024 + 1024 + 1296 + 729$
= $11\ 180$

n = number of Ss or sets of matched Ss
= 10

C = number of conditions
= 3

N = total number or scores, i.e. $n \times C$
= 30

Σx = grand total
= 332

$(\Sigma x)^2$ = grand total squared
= 332^2
= 110224

$\dfrac{(\Sigma x)^2}{N}$ = a constant to be subtracted from all SS
= $\dfrac{110224}{30}$
= 3674.133

x = each individual score

Σx^2 = the sum of each squared individual score
= $15^2 + 12^2 + 11^2 + 12^2 + 9^2 + 8^2 + 13^2 + 10^2 + 11^2 + 10^2 +$
$10^2 + 12^2 + 17^2 + 14^2 + 10^2 + 8^2 + 12^2 + 11^2 + 11^2 + 12^2 +$
$9^2 + 14^2 + 9^2 + 9^2 + 16^2 + 8^2 + 12^2 + 10^2 + 9^2 + 8^2$
= 3840

2. To calculate the SS_{bet}, the formula is:

$$\frac{\Sigma T_c^2}{n} - \frac{(\Sigma x)^2}{N}$$

$$= \frac{126^2 + 105^2 + 101^2}{10} - \frac{110224}{30}$$

$= 3710.2 - 3674.133$
$= 36.067$

3. To calculate the SS_{subj} the formula is:

$$\frac{\Sigma T_s^2}{c} - \frac{(\Sigma x)^2}{N}$$

$$= \frac{38^2 + 29^2 + 34^2 + 32^2 + 41^2 + 31^2 + 32^2 + 32^2 + 36^2 + 27^2}{3} - \frac{110224}{30}$$

$$= 3726.667 - 3674.133$$

$$= 52.534$$

4. To calculate the SS_{tot} the formula is:

$$\Sigma x^2 - \frac{(\Sigma x)^2}{N}$$

$$= 15^2 + 12^2 + 11^2 + 12^2 + 9^2 + 8^2 + 13^2 + 10^2 + 11^2 + 10^2 +$$
$$10^2 + 12^2 + 17^2 + 14^2 + 10^2 + 8^2 + 12^2 + 11^2 + 11^2 + 12^2 +$$
$$9^2 + 14^2 + 9^2 + 9^2 + 16^2 + 8^2 + 12^2 + 10^2 + 9^2 + 8^2 - \frac{110224}{30}$$

$$= 3840 - 3674.133$$

$$= 165.867$$

5. To calculate SS_{error}, the formula is:

$$SS_{tot} - SS_{bet} - SS_{subj}$$

$$= 165.867 - 36.067 - 52.534$$

$$= 77.266$$

6. To calculate the *df values*:

$$
\begin{aligned}
\mathrm{df}_{bet} \quad &= \text{ number of conditions} - 1 \\
&= 3 - 1 \\
&= 2 \\
\mathrm{df}_{subj} \quad &= \text{ number of } Ss - 1 \text{ (or sets of matched } Ss - 1) \\
&= 10 - 1 \\
&= 9 \\
\mathrm{df}_{tot} \quad &= N - 1 \\
&= 30 - 1 \\
&= 29 \\
\mathrm{df}_{error} \quad &= \mathrm{df}_{tot} - \mathrm{df}_{bet} - \mathrm{df}_{subj} \\
&= 29 - 2 - 9 \\
&= 18
\end{aligned}
$$

7. To calculate the *MS* values:

$$
\begin{aligned}
MS_{bet} \quad &= \frac{SS_{bet}}{\mathrm{df}_{bet}} \\[2mm]
&= \frac{36.067}{2} \\[2mm]
&= 18.034
\end{aligned}
$$

$$
\begin{aligned}
MS_{subj} \quad &= \frac{SS_{subj}}{\mathrm{df}_{subj}} \\[2mm]
&= \frac{52.534}{9} \\[2mm]
&= 5.837
\end{aligned}
$$

$$MS_{error} = \frac{SS_{error}}{df_{error}}$$

$$= \frac{77.266}{18}$$

$$= 4.293$$

8. To calculate the F ratios:

F ratio for the *between conditions* variation

$$= \frac{MS_{bet}}{MS_{error}}$$

$$= \frac{18.034}{4.293}$$

$$= 4.201$$

F ratio for the *between subjects* variation

$$= \frac{MS_{subj}}{MS_{error}}$$

$$= \frac{5.837}{4.293}$$

$$= 1.36$$

We can now fill in our table using these values:

Source of variation in scores	Sums of squares SS	Degrees of freedom df	Mean squares MS	F ratios
Variation in scores *between* conditions i.e. aspects of job	36.067	2	18.034	4.201
Variation in scores between *subjects*	52.534	9	5.837	1.36
Variation in scores due to random *error*	77.266	18	4.293	
Total	165.867	29		

Looking up the values of the F ratios

We need to look up these F ratios to find out whether they represent significant differences between the conditions and/or between the subjects. Turn to Tables A2.6a–d which are the probability tables for the anova.

Table a shows the critical values of F at $p < 0.05$.
Table b shows the critical values of F at $p < 0.025$.
Table c shows the critical values of F at $p < 0.01$.
Table d shows the critical values of F at $p < 0.001$.

Note again, that as the anova can only tell us whether there are general differences and *not* whether these differences are in specific direction, these values are for a two-tailed hypothesis.

On each of these Tables you will see that there are values called v_1, across the top and v_2 down the left-hand column. These are df values. To look up the F ratio for the between conditions comparison, we need the df_{bet} value and the df_{error} value. Taking Table a first, locate the df_{bet} (i.e. 2) across the top row, and the df_{error} (i.e. 18) down the left- hand column. Where they intersect is the critical value of F for these df values. If our F ratio of 4.21 is *equal* to or *larger* than the critical value, it is significant at the p value stated at the top of the table. As 4.201 *is* larger than 3.55, we can conclude that our results have an associated probability of less than 5%. But can we do any better? Turn to Table b and repeat the process. Because our value of 4.201 is *smaller* than the intersection value of 4.56 our results are *not* significant at the 0.025 level. Therefore, the probability that our results are due to random error is

less than 0.05

This is expressed, then, as $p < 0.05$.

To find out whether there are differences between the *subjects'* overall performances (i.e. whether the F ratio of 1.36 is significant), we need the df_{subj} value (in this case 9) and the df_{error} value (in this case 18). Look across the v_1 values in Table A2.6a for 9, and down the left-hand column for 18. You will see that there is no v_1 value of 9, so you must take the next smallest. At the intersection point the critical value is 2.51. As our F ratio is *smaller* than this, the results can be said to be not significant. In other words, there is no significant difference between subjects in their overall performance.

Interpreting the results

Our results have an associated probability level of less than 5%, which means that the chances of random error accounting for the results are less than 5 in 100. Since the usual cut-off point is 5%, we can say that our results are significant, which means that the physiotherapists perform some parts of their job better than others. However, the between-subjects F ratio is not significant, which suggests that the physiotherapists concerned did not differ from each other in terms of their overall job performance.

If we take these two results together we can conclude that the senior II physios do indeed perform differently on each aspect of their job, and since there is no significant difference in the overall quality of the physios concerned we may assume that the differences are due to some factor associated with their department, training, attitudes etc. We can express this in the following way:

Using a one-way anova for related subject samples on the data ($F = 4.201$, $N = 10$) it was found that the results were significant at $p < 0.05$. This suggests that there are significant differences in performance levels on the three aspects of the physiotherapist's job investigated. These differences cannot be attributed to variations in the subjects since the F ratio for the between-subjects calculations was not significant ($F = 1.36$, $p = NS$). Therefore, the null hypothesis can be rejected.

It must be remembered that the anova only tells you that there are significant differences between the conditions and not which condition has better/ worse scores. For instance in this example, we know that senior IIs perform differently on three aspects of their job but we do not know whether the difference lies between:

clinical and interpersonal

or

clinical and supervisory

or

interpersonal and supervisory

or

all three.

In order to find out you need to use the Scheffé multiple range test in the next section. However, the Scheffé can *only* be used if the results from the anova are significant.

Activity 26 (Answers on page 284)

1. To practise looking up F ratios, look up the following and state whether or not they are significant and at what level:
   (i) F ratio bet $= 4.96$ $df_{bet} = 2$ $df_{error} = 10$ p
   (ii) F ratio subj $= 4.22$ $df_{subj} = 7$ $df_{error} = 15$ p
   (iii) F ratio subj $= 2.21$ $df_{subj} = 11$ $df_{error} = 20$ p
   (iv) F ratio bet $= 5.15$ $df_{bet} = 14$ $df_{error} = 8$ p
   (v) F ratio subj $= 3.14$ $df_{subj} = 9$ $df_{error} = 14$ p
   (vi) F ratio bet $= 3.98$ $df_{bet} = 10$ $df_{error} = 12$ p
   Remember! Use all the Tables to find the smallest p value possible.
2. Calculate a one-way anova for related designs on the following data:
       H_1 There is a relationship between the type of treatment used on hip replacement patients and the distance walked after 1 week of therapy.
       Brief
       method   Select three groups each of 6 hip replacement patients, matched on age, sex, mobility prior to operation, length of time post- op. etc. Each group is treated using one of three different types of therapy. After 1 week, their mobility is measured in terms of yards walked.

S	Condition A	Condition B	Condition C
	Suspension	Free exercise	Hydrotherapy
1	15	16	11
2	12	14	14
3	10	14	12
4	14	15	12
5	22	19	13
6	17	18	15

State your F ratios, df values and p values in the manner suggested on page 141.

Scheffé multiple range test

The analysis of variance only tells you whether there are *overall* differences between the conditions and not where these differences lie. As a result, it is not possible from this test alone to conclude whether the scores from one condition are significantly better or worse than those from another. If you look back to the example given, the anova only allows us to conclude that physiotherapists perform *differently* in aspects of their job — it does not permit us to say that their performance on one task is better than their performance on another. However, if you look at the results for each condition (p. 135) it appears that the Clinical scores are better than the Interpersonal scores, with the Supervisory scores being worst. We can find out whether the differences between these sets of results are significant by comparing each pair of mean scores using the Scheffé multiple range test. In other words, we can compare:

1. the mean Clinical score with the mean Interpersonal score
2. the mean Clinical score with the mean Supervisory score
3. the mean Interpersonal score with the mean Supervisory score.

to find out if the differences in performance in each area are significant. The Scheffé test should be carried out *after* you have calculated the anova because it uses some of the values from the anova table. Remember, too, that it should be carried out *only* if the results from the anova are significant.

There are a number of other multiple range tests which perform the same function, but the Scheffé has been selected because it is considered to be the best (McNemar, 1963) and also because it can be used if there are unequal numbers of subjects in each condition. Obviously this latter point does not apply in same subject and matched subject designs (since you will, by definition, have the same number of scores in each condition) but since the Scheffé can also be used with a one-way anova for unrelated designs and unequal subject numbers this feature is a useful one.

When calculating the Scheffé, you find two values. Firstly, F is calculated for each comparison of means you wish to make, and secondly F^1 is calculated. Each F is compared with the F^1 value. If it is equal to or larger than the F^1 value, then the result is significant.

Calculating the Scheffé

There are three possible comparisons we can make using the Scheffé on our sample data:

1. Clinical vs Interpersonal Scores
2. Clinical vs Supervisory Scores
3. Interpersonal vs Supervisory Scores.

To make these comparisons, take the following steps:
1. Calculate the mean score for each condition
$$\bar{x}_1 = 12.6; \qquad \bar{x}_2 = 10.5; \qquad \bar{x}_3 = 10.1$$
2. Find the value of F for the first comparison (i.e. Clinical vs Interpersonal) using the following formula:

$$F = \frac{(\bar{x}_1 - \bar{x}_2)^2}{\dfrac{MS_{subj}}{n_1} + \dfrac{MS_{subj}}{n_2}}$$

where $\bar{x}_1$ = mean for *Condition 1*
           = 12.6
$\bar{x}_2$ = mean for *Condition 2*
           = 10.5
MS_{subj} = mean square value for the *between subjects* variation (from the anova calculations)
           = 5.837
n_1 = number of subjects in *Condition 1*
           = 10
n_2 = number of subjects in *Condition 2*
           = 10

If these values are substituted, then

$$F = \frac{(12.6 - 10.5)^2}{\dfrac{5.837}{10} + \dfrac{5.837}{10}}$$

$$= \frac{4.41}{1.168}$$

$$= 3.776$$

3. Repeat the calculations for the other two comparisons, using the appropriate means and n values.

∴ for the comparison of the Clinical and Supervisory scores, the formula is:

$$F = \frac{(\bar{x}_1 - \bar{x}_3)^2}{\dfrac{MS_{subj}}{n_1} + \dfrac{MS_{subj}}{n_3}}$$

$$= \frac{(12.6 - 10.1)^2}{\dfrac{5.837}{10} + \dfrac{5.837}{10}}$$

$$= 5.351$$

and for the comparison of the Interpersonal and Supervisory scores, the formula is:

$$F = \frac{(\bar{x}_2 - \bar{x}_3)^2}{\dfrac{MS_{subj}}{n_2} + \dfrac{MS_{subj}}{n_3}}$$

$$= \frac{(10.5 - 10.1)^2}{\dfrac{5.837}{10} + \dfrac{5.837}{10}}$$

$$= 0.137$$

4. Using the df_{bet} and df_{subj} values derived from the anova (i.e. 2 and 9 respectively), turn to Table A2.6a and locate the df_{bet} value across the v_1 row, and the df_{subj} down the v_2 column. At the intersection point, you will find the value of 4.26. This is the critical value for F at the $<$ 5% or < 0.05 level of significance. The < 5% level is selected because of the extreme stringency of the Scheffé test. If a smaller p value were to be selected, you would be far less likely to obtain significant results on the Scheffé. However, should you ever get any results that look as though they are considerably more significant than the 5% level, you can repeat steps 4–6 with Tables A2.6b (1%), A2.6c (2½%) and A2.6d (0.1%).

5. Calculate F^1 using the formula

$$(C - 1) F^\circ$$

where C = the number of conditions
            = 3
            F° = the figure at the intersection point of the appropriate df values in Table
            = 4.26

$$F^1 = (3 - 1)\,4.26$$
$$= 8.52$$

6. Compare the F values derived from the calculations in steps 2 and 3 with the F^1 value above. If the F value is *equal* to or *larger* than the F^1 value it is significant.

Therefore, taking our F values of

     3.776
     5.351
     0.137

we can see that they are *all* smaller than the F^1 value and so none is significant. Therefore, there are no significant differences between pairs of conditions.

Interpreting the results

The results from the Scheffé test indicate that there are no significant differences between pairs of performance scores. This is interesting because the anova produced a significant overall difference between the conditions ($p < 0.05$). How can these conflicting results be reconciled? Firstly, the Scheffé is a very stringent test and leads to fewer significant results than other multiple range tests. But, secondly, these results indicate that while there are general overall differences in performance for each aspect of the job, no one pair of scores is responsible for this. Instead the results from the anova are the product of the contributions made from an interaction of *all* the differences in scores. So, we can conclude that there are overall differences in performance, but no one aspect of the job is carried out significantly better or worse than any other. Had we found significant differences (say, between the Clinical and the Supervisory scores) we could conclude that the results are significant at the < 5% level (since we used the < 5% table to calculate F) and that this difference is a major, though not sole, contributor to the overall differences found by the anova. (Remember, the Table for the < 5% level of significance is used to calculate the F value as a rule, since, because the Scheffé is so stringent; if the 1% and 0.1% tables were used, we'd very rarely obtain significant results!)

Activity 27 (Answers on page 285)

Carry out a Scheffé test on the following results:

H_1 There is a difference in the efficacy of four teaching approaches used with student physiotherapists.

Method A group of 15 student physiotherapists are given comparable information in four different ways — seminar, tutorial, lecture, and individual reading. They are tested on their understanding and receive marks out of 20. A one-way anova for related designs was computed on the scores and the following relevant results obtained:

$$df_{bet} = 3$$
$$df_{subj} = 14$$
$$MS_{subj} = 3.87$$

The mean scores for each condition were

Condition 1 Seminar 11.2
Condition 2 Tutorial 13.1
Condition 3 Lecture 10.7
Condition 4 Reading 8.4

9

Non-parametric tests for different (unrelated) subject designs

The statistical tests described in this chapter are used when the experimental design involves two or more than two *different* unmatched groups of subjects who are compared on a certain task, activity etc. All the tests covered in this chapter are non-parametric ones, which means that they

— are less sensitive
— are easier to calculate
— can be used on nominal, ordinal or interval/ratio data.

Therefore, if you cannot fulfil the conditions required for parametric tests, you should use its non-parametric equivalent.

The designs involved in this chapter, then, are:

1. Two different, unmatched subject groups compared on a certain task, activity etc.

Subject group 1 takes part in *Condition 1*   ⎫ Results from conditions are
Subject group 2 takes part in *Condition 2*   ⎭ compared for differences

or

2. Three or more different, unmatched subject groups compared on a certain task, activity etc.

Subject group 1 takes part in *Condition 1*   ⎫
Subject group 2 takes part in *Condition 2*   ⎬ Results from conditions are compared for differences
Subject group 3 takes part in *Condition 3*   ⎭

Results from Design 1 are analysed using the Chi-squared (χ^2) test if the data is nominal or the Mann-Whitney U test if it is other than nominal (i.e. ordinal or interval/ratio).

Results from Design 2 are analysed using the Extended Chi-squared (χ^2) test if the data is nominal or the Kruskal-Wallis test if the data is other than nominal (i.e. ordinal or interval/ratio). If a trend in the results is predicted, such that subject group a is expected to perform better than subject group b, with subject group c performing worst, the Jonckheere trend test is used as long as the data is other than nominal.

Table 9.1 Tests for different subjects designs

Design	Non parametric test
1. Two different groups of subjects, compared on a task.	Chi-squared test if data is nominal Mann-Whitney U test (if data is other than nominal, i.e. ordinal or interval/ratio).
2. Three or more different groups of subjects, compared on a task.	Extended Chi-squared test if data is nominal. Kruskal-Wallis (if just a difference in results is predicted and the data is other than nominal, i.e. ordinal or interval/ratio). Jonckheere trend test (if a trend in the results is predicted and the data is other than nominal, i.e. ordinal or interval/ratio).

NON-PARAMETRIC STATISTICAL TEST FOR USE WITH TWO DIFFERENT SUBJECT GROUPS AND NOMINAL DATA

Chi-squared (χ^2) test

This test is used when you have the sort of experimental design which uses two different unmatched groups of subjects who are compared on a task, activity etc. The data for the χ^2 test (pronounced Kie-squared) must be *nominal*.

To refresh your memory, the nominal level of measurement only allows you to allocate your subjects to named categories (e.g. pass/fail; Asian/West Indian/Caucasian; good/bad; mobile/immobile) — it does not allow you to measure your subjects' responses, i.e. how well they have passed, how mobile they are. Check Chapter 5 to make sure you're happy with this concept. As you can see, a subject may only be allocated to one category, since it is impossible to be both mobile *and* immobile, to pass *and* to fail. Because of this the χ^2 can *only* be used when *different* subjects are allocated to *different* categories, i.e. an unrelated design.

With the χ^2 test you may only use *two* nominal categories and *two* subject groups. For example you may wish to find out whether there is a difference between men and women in terms of which hip (left or right) is more likely to be replaced. You have *two* groups:

men and women

and two nominal categories:

left and right

Should you ever wish to allocate *two* groups to *more than two* nominal categories you must use the *Extended* χ^2 (see p. 168).

It should also be noted that when you use the χ^2 test, you should ensure that *at least* 20 subjects will be in each group. While this may sound off-putting, it rarely takes too much time to collect this amount of data.

What the χ^2 test does is to compare the numbers *obtained* in the experiment for each nominal category with the numbers which could be *expected by chance* to see if the differences between them are sufficiently great to be classified as significant. The numbers obtained in the experiment are referred to as *observed frequencies*, while the numbers which are expected by chance are called *expected frequencies*. When you calculate the χ^2 test, you find a numerical value for χ^2 which you then look up in the probability tables associated with the χ^2 test to see if this value represents a significant difference between the result you observed and those that could be expected by chance.

Example

Let's suppose you were interested in the effects of encouraging early weight bearing after ligamentous ankle sprain. Your hypothesis is:

H_1 Patients who are encouraged to bear full weight after ligamentous ankle sprains are more likely to achieve an early restoration of normal gait pattern.

Method You select 30 sprained ankle patients and give them full weight bearing exercises for 15 minutes each day. A further 32 sprained ankle patients are given no exercise. After 3 days, you assess the gait pattern for each group. You count up how many patients have a normal gait pattern and how many do not.

This is a *nominal* level of measurement because you are using two categories — 'normal gait pattern' and 'abnormal gait pattern' and are simply allocating subjects to one of these groups.

You have a design which looks like this:

Subject group 1 30 sprained ankle patients	takes part in	*Condition 1* Full weight bearing exercises	Assessed as to whether they have normal gait pattern after 3 days. The results are compared.
Subject group 2 32 sprained ankle patients	takes part in	*Condition 2* No weight-bearing exercises	

In other words you have *two* groups of subjects who can be allocated to *two* nominal categories (normal gait pattern or not.)

You end up with the following results:

	Normal gait pattern	Abnormal gait pattern	Marginal totals
Subject group 1 Exercises	A 21	B 9	A + B 30
Subject group 2 No exercises	C 14	D 18	C + D 32
Marginal totals	A + C 35	B + D 27	Grand total N 62

Calculating the χ^2 test

1. The first step you must always take is to set your data out in a 2 × 2 table as shown above. The subject groups should go down the side and the nominal categories across the top, although it doesn't matter which category is on the left, nor which subject group is at the top. Label your Cells A, B, C, and D in the *same way* as above (i.e. from left to right).
2. You must now add up the marginal totals for each row and each column
   i.e. A + B = 21 + 9
   $\qquad$ = 30
   $\quad$ C + D = 14 + 18
   $\qquad$ = 32
   $\quad$ A + C = 21 + 14
   $\qquad$ = 35
   $\quad$ B + D = 9 + 18
   $\qquad$ = 27
3. Calculate the Grand total N *either* by adding up the vertical marginal totals
   i.e. 30 + 32
   = 62
   or by adding up the horizontal marginal totals
   i.e. 35 + 27
   = 62
   (The answer will be the same.)
4. Find χ^2 from the formula

$$\chi^2 = \frac{N \left[(AD - BC) - \dfrac{N}{2} \right]^2}{(A + B)(C + D)(A + C)(B + D)}$$

$\quad$ where N = the Grand total, i.e. 62
$\qquad$ AD = Cell A × Cell D = 21 × 18
$\qquad\qquad\qquad\qquad\quad$ = 378
$\qquad$ BC = Cell B × Cell C = 9 × 14
$\qquad\qquad\qquad\qquad\quad$ = 126

The values under the division line are all the marginal totals:

$A + B = 30$
$C + D = 32$
$A + C = 35$
$B + D = 27$

Therefore, if we substitute these values in the formula:

$$\chi^2 = \frac{62 \left[(378 - 126^*) - \frac{62}{2} \right]^2}{30 \times 32 \times 35 \times 27}$$

$$= \frac{3028142}{907200}$$

$$\chi^2 = 3.338$$

(*If you get a minus number from the calculations in the inner brackets, ignore the minus sign)

5. Before this χ^2 value can be looked up in the probability tables to see if it represents a significant difference, the df value is required. Using the df formula of:

$$(r - 1)(c - 1)$$

where r = the number of rows
       c = the number of columns
         = $(2 - 1)(2 - 1)$
         = 1

Obviously, in a 2×2 table like this, the df will *always* equal 1.

Looking up the value of χ^2 for significance

To find out whether the χ^2 value of 3.338 represents a significant difference in gait pattern between patients who have done full weight bearing exercise and those who have not, it must be looked up in the probability tables associated with the χ^2 test (Table A2.1).

Down the left-hand column you will see df values from 1–30. Look down this column until you find the df value of 1. To the right of this are five numbers, called *critical values* of χ^2:

2.71   3.84   5.41   6.64   10.83.

Each of these critical values is associated with the probability level at the top of its column, e.g. the critical value of 5.41 is associated with 0.02 for a two-tailed test. You will see that the p values in the table are only associated with two-tailed hypotheses. If you have a one-tailed hypothesis, simply look up your χ^2 value as described, find the two-tailed p value and *halve* it (see pp 98–99).

In order for our χ^2 value of 3.338 to be significant at one of these levels, it has to be *equal to* or *larger than* one of these numbers. Our value is larger than 2.71 but smaller than 3.84. Therefore, we must select the critical value of 2.71 (remember our χ^2 must be equal to or larger). This is associated with a probability level of 0.10 for a two-tailed test and therefore 0.05 for a one-tailed test (i.e. *half* 0.10). As our hypothesis predicted a specific direction to the results (full weight bearing exercises are *more* likely to lead to normal gait pattern), our results are associated with a p value of 0.05.

Now because our χ^2 value is *larger* than the critical value of 2.71, this means the p value is actually *less than* 0.05. This is expressed as

$$p < 0.05$$

This means that the probability of our results being due to random error is less than 5%.

Interpreting the results

Our χ^2 value has an associated probability level of less than 0.05 or 5%, which means that the chance of random error being responsible for the results is less than 5%. Because a 5% cut-off point is usually used to claim that the results support the experimental hypothesis, we can say that our results are significant.

However, before we can finally conclude that the hypothesis has been supported, just go back to the 2 × 2 table and check the results are in the predicted direction, because it is quite possible sometimes to obtain significant results which are *opposite* to those predicted in the hypothesis and so would *not* support the hypothesis.

Here we find that more of the exercise group have a normal gait pattern (21 vs 14) and more of the non-exercise group have an abnormal gait pattern (18 vs 9). Therefore the results are as predicted. We can reject the null (no difference) hypothesis on this basis. This can be expressed in the following way:

Using a χ^2 test on the data ($\chi^2 = 3.338$, df = 1) the results were found to be significant at $p < 0.05$, for a one-tailed test. This suggests that the null hypothesis can be rejected and that patients who are encouraged to bear full weight after ligamentous ankle sprain are more likely to achieve an early restoration of normal gait pattern.

Activity 28 (Answers on page 285)
1. In order to practise looking up χ^2 values, look up the following and say what the associated p value is and whether or not it is significant.
   (i) $\chi^2 = 4.02$ one-tailed   df = 1 p
   (ii) $\chi^2 = 5.91$ two-tailed   df = 1 p
   (iii) $\chi^2 = 3.84$ two-tailed   df = 1 p
   (iv) $\chi^2 = 2.62$ two-tailed   df = 1 p
   (v) $\chi^2 = 6.95$ one-tailed   df = 1 p

2. Calculate a χ^2 test on the following.

H_1 Teachers of physiotherapy are more likely to study in Open University degree courses than clinically-based physiotherapists of comparable years of experience since qualifying.

Method   You randomly select 35 teachers of physiotherapy and 40 clinically-based physiotherapists and ask them whether or not they have ever undertaken an OU degree course.

The results are as follows:

	OU course	No OU course
Teachers of physiotherapy	25	10
Clinically-based physiotherapists	15	27

State your χ^2 value, p value, using the sample format given on page 152.

NON-PARAMETRIC STATISTICAL TEST FOR USE WITH TWO DIFFERENT, UNMATCHED SUBJECT GROUPS AND ORDINAL OR INTERVAL/RATIO DATA

Mann-Whitney U test

This test is used to analyse results from experiments which have compared two different, unmatched groups of subjects on a task (see Design 1, page 147). The Mann-Whitney U test simply compares the results from each group to see if they differ significantly. This test can only be used with ordinal or interval/ratio data. It cannot be used with nominal data.

When calculating this test, you end up with a numerical value for U which you look up in the probability tables associated with the Mann-Whitney test, to see if the U value does, in fact, represent a significant difference between the groups.

Example

Suppose you were interested in testing the hypothesis that there is a difference in the rate of healing of non-infected bed-scores among bed-ridden geriatrics when treated by infrared or ice-cube massage.

Your hypothesis would be:

H_1 There is a difference in the healing rates of non-infected bed-sores of bed-ridden geriatric patients when treated by infrared as opposed to ice-cube massage.

In order to do this, you select a group of 28 elderly patients, all of whom have non-infected bed-sores. (Assume constant errors have been eliminated, e.g. length of time bed-ridden.) Randomly allocate 15 patients to infrared and 13 to ice-cube massage.

Therefore, we have the following design:

Group 1 15 elderly patients	treated by	Condition 1 Infrared	The two groups are compared for extent of healing (e.g. on a 9-point scale where 9 = totally healed, 1 = not at all healed).
Group 2 13 elderly patients	treated by	Condition 2 Ice-cube massage	

Essentially, you would administer different treatments to each group and compare the extent of the healing after a given period of time, e.g. 7 days. (Note that because we don't have to match the subjects, you can use different numbers in each group.) You might end up with the following results:

Subject	Condition 1 Infrared	Rank	Subject	Condition 2 Ice-cube massage	Rank
1	6	18	1	7	22.5
2	5	12.5	2	9	27.5
3	7	22.5	3	6	18
4	3	2.5	4	5	12.5
5	5	12.5	5	6	18
6	4	7	6	7	22.5
7	4	7	7	7	22.5
8	3	2.5	8	8	25.5
9	8	25.5	9	9	27.5
10	6	18	10	6	18
11	5	12.5	11	5	12.5
12	4	7	12	4	7
13	3	2.5	13	5	12.5
14	3	2.5			
15	4	7			
Total	70	159.5		84	246.5
Mean	4.667			6.462	

Calculating the Mann-Whitney U test

To calculate the Mann-Whitney, take the following steps:
1. First calculate the totals (Σ) and means for each condition:
   i.e. *Condition 1* Total : 70
   Mean : 4.667
   Condition 2 Total : 84
   Mean : 6.462
2. Taking the *whole set of scores* together (i.e. all 28 scores) rank them

giving the rank of 1 to the lowest, 2 to the next lowest and so on. Where there are 2 or more scores the same, use the tied rank procedure (see pp 112–113), i.e. add up the ranks the scores would have obtained had they been different and divide this number by the number of scores that are the same. Thus 3 is the lowest score, but there are four scores of 3. Therefore add up the ranks 1, 2, 3 and 4 (the ranks they would have obtained had they been different) and divide by 4 because there are *4* scores of 3.

i.e. $\dfrac{1 + 2 + 3 + 4}{4} = 2.5$

Assign the rank of 2.5 to all the scores of 3. (See columns labelled rank.) Remember! Put the scores from both conditions *together*, as though they were just *one* set of scores, when you do the ranking. Many students forget to do this.

3. Add the rank totals for each condition separately.
    i.e. Rank total 1 = 159.5
       Rank total 2 = 246.5
4. Select the *larger* rank total, i.e. 246.5 to use in the formula below.
5. Find U from the formula:
    $$U = n_1 n_2 + \frac{n_x (n_x + 1)}{2} - T_x$$

Where n_1 = the number of subjects in *Condition 1* (i.e. 15)
    n_2 = the number of subjects in *Condition 2* (i.e. 13)
    T_x = the larger rank total (i.e. 246.5)
    n_x = the number of Ss in the condition with the larger rank total
       (I.e. Condition 2 = 13)

∴ if we substitute these values
    $$U = 15 \times 13 + \frac{13 (13 + 1)}{2} - 246.5$$
    $$= 195 + 91 - 246.5$$
    $$= 39.5$$

6. Because there are *unequal* numbers in each condition, it is necessary to repeat the calculations for the smaller rank total (i.e. 159.5) as well. Here T_x becomes the smaller rank total (159.5)
    and n_x becomes the number of subjects in the condition with the smaller rank total (i.e. *Conditon 1* = 15 subjects).
    $$U_2 = 15 \times 13 + \frac{15 (15 + 1)}{2} - 159.5$$
    $$= 195 + 120 - 159.5$$
    $$= 155.5$$

We now have two values of U:
    $$U = 39.5$$
    $$U_2 = 155.5$$

We need to look up the *smaller* of these two U values in the appropriate table (A2.7a–d).

Note that if you use *equal* numbers of subjects in each condition, you only need to carry out the first calculation of U, using the *larger* rank total and the appropriate n value. If you use unequal numbers you will have to find *both* U values and select the *smaller* one.

Looking up the value of U for significance

In order to find out whether our U value of 39.5 represents a significant difference in healing rates, you have to look up this value in Tables A2.7a–d. There are *four* probability tables for the Mann-Whitney, each one representing different p values (see headings). Table A2.7a represents the smallest (most significant) p values. While Table A2.7d represents the largest (least significant) p value. To look up your U value you also need:

$$n_1 \text{ value (15)}$$
$$n_2 \text{ value (13)}$$

Starting with Table A2.7a, look across the top row until you find your n_1 value of 15, and down the left-hand column for your n_2 value of 13. Where these two points intersect is the number 42. In order to be significant at a given level, your U value must be *equal* to or *smaller* than the value at the intersection point. As 39.5 *is* smaller than 42, our results are significant at either 0.005 for a one-tailed test or 0.01 for a two-tailed test. As we only predicted a *general* difference in healing rates in our hypothesis without specifying which treatment would be better, we have a two-tailed hypothesis. Therefore, our results are significant at the 0.01 or 1% probability level. *But*, if you notice, our U value of 39.5 is actually *smaller* than the value of 42 at the intersection point. This means our results are significant at *even less* than the 1% level. This is expressed as:

$$p < 0.01 \text{ or } < 1\%$$

Had our U value been the same as the value at the intersection point, the results would have been significant at *exactly* the 0.01 or 1% level. This would have been expressed as:

$$p = 0.01 \text{ (or 1\%)}$$

However, our results have a probabiliy of *less* than 1% which means that the chance of random error accounting for our results is less than 1%.

Supposing, however, our U value had been 52.5, with our n values the same. Using A2.7a, we would find that the intersection value is 42. Because our U of 52.5 is *larger* than this value, it would not be significant at the probability levels of 0.005 and 0.01 given in the heading. Therefore, we would move on to Table A2.7b. At this intersection point for $n_1 = 15$, $n_2 = 13$, the value is 47. Our U value is *larger* than this and so cannot be classified as significant at this level either. Turn on to Table A2.7c. The intersection value here is 54. Our U value is *smaller* and so would be significant at the < 0.05 level for a two-tailed test.

If you ever find your U value is larger than the relevant intersection values in Table A2.7d, your results would not be significant.

Interpreting the results

Our U value has an associated probability level of less than 1% which means that there is less than a 1% chance of random error causing the results. If you remember, it was said that a good cut-off point for claiming that your results were significant and supported your hypothesis was the 5% level or less. Since our p value is less than 5% we can claim our results are significant; our null (no relationship) hypothesis can therefore be rejected and the experimental hypothesis supported.

Although the hypothesis did not predict which of the two treatments would be better, it is useful to compare the means from each condition to see which method was, in fact, more successful. Here the mean scores are 4.667 and 6.462 for infrared and ice-cube massage respectively, which means that ice-cube massage was more effective. This can be stated in the following way:

Using a Mann-Whitney U test to analyse that data ($U = 39.5$, $n_1 = 15$, $n_2 = 13$), the results were found to be significant at $p < 0.01$ for a two-tailed hypothesis. This means that infrared treatment and ice-cube massage differ significantly in their effectiveness in treating non-infected bed-sores in elderly bed-ridden patients. Futher inspection of the results suggest that ice-cube massage produces better results.

Activity 29 (Answers on pages 285–286)

1. To practise looking up U values, look up the following and state whether or not they're significant and at what level.

   (i) $n = 12$ $n = 12$ $U = 33.5$ two-tailed p
   (ii) $n = 10$ $n = 10$ $U = 27$ one-tailed p
   (iii) $n = 14$ $n = 12$ $U = 37.5$ one-tailed p
   (iv) $n = 20$ $n = 18$ $U = 87.5$ one-tailed p
   (v) $n = 15$ $n = 15$ $U = 70.5$ one-tailed p
   (vi) $n = 18$ $n = 15$ $U = 92.5$ two-tailed p

2. Calculate a Mann-Whitney U test on the following:

   H_1 Paraffin wax is more effective than a hot soak as a preparation for mobilising exercises for post-fracture patients.

   Method   Randomly select 28 patients all of whom are within 1 week post removal of plaster following forearm fracture. Randomly allocate 14 to paraffin wax treatment and the other 14 to a hot soak. Rate the ease of movement of the wrist joint following 30 minutes of mobilising exercises on a 7 point scale (7 = extremely easy to move, 1 = very difficult to move).

Subject	Condition 1 Paraffin wax	Rank	Subject	Condition 2 Hot soak	Rank
1	5		1	3	
2	4		2	3	
3	5		3	5	
4	6		4	4	
5	3		5	2	
6	3		6	1	
7	4		7	3	
8	5		8	4	
9	6		9	5	
10	5		10	5	
11	6		11	3	
12	6		12	3	
13	4		13	4	
14	3		14	2	

State the U value and the p value in a format similar to that suggested earlier.

NON-PARAMETRIC STATISTICAL TESTS FOR USE WITH THREE OR MORE DIFFERENT, UNMATCHED SUBJECT GROUPS AND ORDINAL OR INTERVAL/RATIO DATA

1. Kruskal-Wallis test

This test is simply an extension of the Mann-Whitney test, in that it is used:

— when different subject groups are involved
— when the data is ordinal, or interval/ratio
— when the conditions for its parametric equivalent cannot be fulfilled.

However, while the Mann-Whitney can only be used to analyse the results from designs with *two* different groups of subjects, the Kruskal-Wallis is used with designs employing *3 or more* different groups of subjects:

Subject group 1 $\dfrac{\text{takes part}}{\text{in}}$ *Condition 1*

Subject group 2 $\dfrac{\text{takes part}}{\text{in}}$ *Condition 2*

Subject group 3 (etc.) $\dfrac{\text{takes part}}{\text{in}}$ *Condition 3*

Compare results from the groups to see if there are differences between them

The Kruskal-Wallis, however, only tells you whether there *are* differences between these groups and not which results are better or worse than the others. Therefore, the associated hypothesis must be two-tailed (i.e. just predicting differences in the results with no specific direction to them). Should you ever predict a *trend* in your results, e.g. that Group a will perform better than Group b, which in turn will perform better than Group c with this sort of unrelated design, you would use a Jonckheere trend test to analyse your results.

However, with the Kruskal-Wallis, you calculate the value of H, which you then look up in the probability tables associated with the Kruskal-Wallis test, to find out whether the H value represents significant differences between the groups.

Example

Let's suppose you are working with stroke patients and are trying to help them regain the use of paralysed limbs. You always give the patients some preparatory warm-up exercises, but would be interested to see whether some of these preparations are more effective than others. So you decide to compare the effectiveness of three preparatory procedures on the contraction of the biceps.

Your hypothesis, then, is:

H$_1$ There is difference in the strength of muscle contraction in the biceps, according to whether it is preceded by 2 minutes infrared radiation, 2 minutes specific warm-up or 2 minutes general warm-up.

In order to test this out, you select 30 stroke patients and randomly allocate them to one of the three groups. Following the 2 minutes selected preparation you rate the strength of their biceps contraction on a 5-point scale (5 = very strong, 1 = very weak).

Your design looks like this:

Subject group 1 10 Stroke patients	takes part —————— in	*Condition 1* Infrared	
Subject group 2 10 Stroke patients	takes part —————— in	*Condition 2* Specific warm-up	Groups compared for differences in muscle contraction
Subject group 3 10 Stroke patients	takes part —————— in	*Condition 3* General warm-up	

Your results look like this:

Subject*	Condition 1 Infrared	Rank	Subject	Condition 2 Specific	Rank	Subject	Condition 3 General	Rank
1	3	16	1	4	24	1	2	8
2	4	24	2	5	29	2	3	16
3	2	8	3	5	29	3	3	16
4	2	8	4	4	24	4	4	24
5	1	2.5	5	4	24	5	1	2.5
6	3	16	6	3	16	6	3	16
7	4	24	7	2	8	7	2	8
8	1	2.5	8	3	16	8	1	2.5
9	2	8	9	5	29	9	3	16
10	2	8	10	4	24	10	3	16
Total	24	117.0		39	223		25	125.0
Mean	2.4			3.9			2.5	

* Because this is a different, unmatched subject design, you do not have to have equal numbers of subjects in each group, although it is easier if you do.

Calculating the Kruskal-Wallis

1. Calculate the Totals and Mean scores for each condition:
   Condition 1 Total = 24 $\bar{x} = 2.4$
   Condition 2 Total = 39 $\bar{x} = 3.9$
   Condition 3 Total = 25 $\bar{x} = 2.5$.
2. Taking *all* the scores together, as though they were a single set of 30 scores, rank the scores, giving a rank of 1 to the lowest score, a rank of 2 to the next lowest etc. Where 2 or more scores are the same, apply the average ranks procedure (see pp 112–113), i.e. add up the ranks the scores would have obtained had they been different and divide this number by the total number of scores that are the same. Thus, in the example, 1 is the lowest score, but there are *4* scores of 1. Had these been different, they would have been ranked 1, 2, 3 and 4. So add these ranks up (10) and divide by *4* because there were *four* scores of 1 (i.e. 2.5). Give the rank of 2.5 to all the scores of 1. Remember that you have now used up ranks 1–4, so you must start with 5 next.
   Remember! Rank all the scores together, as though they were just one set of 30 scores.
3. Add the rank total for each condition separately to give *T*:
   $T_c1 = 117.0$
   $T_c2 = 223$
   $T_c3 = 125.0$.
4. Find the value of H from the following formula:

$$H = \left[\frac{12}{N(N+1)} \left(\sum \frac{T_c^2}{n_c} \right) \right] - 3(N+1)$$

where N = total number of subjects (i.e. 30)
   n_c = number of subjects in each group
      (i.e. $n_1 = 10$; $n_2 = 10$; $n_3 = 10$)
   T_c = rank totals for each condition
      (i.e. $T_c1 = 117$; $T_c2 = 223$; $T_c3 = 125$)
   T_c^2 = rank total for each condition *squared*
      (i.e. 117^2; 223^2; 125^2)
   Σ = total of any calculations following

$$\sum \frac{T_c^2}{n_c}$$ = the number of the rank totals squared divided by the
   number of subjects in that condition

   i.e. $\dfrac{117^2}{10} + \dfrac{223^2}{10} + \dfrac{125^2}{10}$

Substituting these values:

$$H = \left[\frac{12}{30\,(30 + 1)} \times \left(\frac{117^2}{10} + \frac{223^2}{10} + \frac{125^2}{10} \right) \right] - 3 \times 31$$

$$= \left[\frac{12}{930} \times (1368.9 + 4972.9 + 1562.5) \right] - 93$$

$$= (0.013 \times 7904.3) - 93$$
$$= 102.756 - 93$$
$$= 9.756$$

Looking up the H value for significance

To find out whether $H = 9.756$ represents significant differences between the results from each group, you will also need the df value. This is the number of conditions minus 1, i.e. $3 - 1 = 2$. Turn to Tables A2.1 and A2.8. Table A2.8 covers the probability levels for experiments using three groups of subjects, with 1–5 subjects in each group, while Table A2.1 covers the probabilty levels for experiments with more subjects and more conditions. (This is also the Chi-squared table.)

Because we have 10 subjects in each condition we use Table A2.1. Down the left-hand column you will see various df values. Look down the column until you find out df of 2. To the right of this are 5 numbers:

   4.60   5.99   7.82   9.21   13.82

These are called *critical values* and each one is associated with the probability level indicated at the top of the column, e.g. 7.82 has a p value of 0.02. To be significant at a given level, our H value has to be *equal* to or *larger* than one of these numbers. So, with our H of 9.756, we can see that it is larger than 9.21, but *smaller* than 13.82. Therefore, we must select the value of 9.21 (because our H value is *larger* than 9.21). If you look up this column, you will see that this indicates a significance level of 0.01 or 1%. (Remember there are only two-tailed p values, because with the Kruskal-

Wallis, we can only predict general differences in our results.) However, because our H value is *larger* than the critical value of 9.21, the probability level is even *less* than 0.01. This is expressed as $p < 0.01$ or $< 1\%$. This means that there is less than a 1% chance that our results are due to random error. (Had our H value been *equal* to the critical value, p would have been 0.01 *exactly*. This would have been expressed as $p = 0.01$ or 1%.)

Interpreting the results

Our H value of 9.756 has a probability of < 0.01 (or $< 1\%$) which means that the probability of random error accounting for the results is less than 1%. As you will remember, it was noted earlier that the usual cut-off point for assuming support for the experimental hypothesis is the 5% level or less. As our p value is less than 1%, it is smaller than the cut-off point of 5% and therefore we can say that our results are significant. This means we can *reject* the null hypothesis and accept the experimental hypothesis. This can be expressed in the following way:

> Using a Kruskal-Wallis test on the data ($H = 9.756$, $N = 30$) the results were found to be significant at $p < 0.01$. This suggests that there is a significant difference in the strength of muscle contractions with different preparation techniques among stroke patients. This means that the experimental hypothesis has been supported.

Remember that the Kruskal-Wallis will only tell you that there are differences between your conditions and not which preparation is most effective. If you had hypothesised a *trend* in the results, e.g.

specific warm-up is better than general warm-up which in turn is better than infrared

and had used the same unmatched design, you would used a Jonckheere trend test to analyse your results (see p. 163).

Because we used more than 5 Ss in our experiment, we had to use Table A2.1 to look up our H value. Suppose, however, that we had used instead, 5 Ss in *Condition 1*, 4 in *Condition 2* and 3 in *Condition 3*, and had obtained an H value of 5.438. We would now need to use Table A2.8. You will see that there is a heading 'Size of groups', under which there is every permutation of n values. Your n values are $n_1 = 5$, $n_2 = 4$ and $n_3 = 3$. Therefore you need to find these n values (in any order) in the columns and to the right of these you will see six values of H:

7.4449
7.3949
5.6564
5.6308
4.5487
4.5231

and to their right, the relevant p values. (You do not need the df value here.)

To be significant at a given level, our H value must be *equal* to or *larger* than the critical values here. Our hypothesised H value of 5.438 is larger than 4.5231 and 4.5487 but smaller than 5.6308. Therefore we must take the next smallest value — 4.54487 — which is associated with a p value of 0.099. Because our cut-off point is 0.05, we must accept the null (no relationship) hypothesis, i.e. our results would not be significant.

Activity 30 (Answers on page 286)

1. To practise looking up H values, look up the following and state whether or not they are signficant and at what level.

   (i) $n_1 = 3$ $n_2 = 4$ $n_3 = 3$ $H = 5.801$ p
   (ii) $n_1 = 5$ $n_2 = 5$ $n_3 = 4$ $H = 5.893$ p
   (iii) $n_1 = 12$ $n_2 = 10$ $n_3 = 10$ $n_4 = 10$ df $= 3$ $H = 8.5$ p
   (iv) $n_1 = 3$ $n_2 = 3$ $n_3 = 5$ $H = 7.0234$ p
   (v) $n_1 = 10$ $n_2 = 12$ $n_3 = 14$ $n_4 = 14$
      $n_5 = 14$ df $= 4$ $H = 15.23$ p
   (vi) $n_1 = 10$ $n_2 = 10$ $n_3 = 8$ $n_4 = 10$ df $= 3$ $H = 6.86$ p

2. Calculate a Kruskal-Wallis on the following data:

   H_1 Compliance with postnatal exercise instructions varies according to whether the instructions are (a) oral, (b) written by the physiotherapist or (c) written by the patient herself.

   Method   Select 15 women within 1 week of parturition and randomly allocate 5 to oral instructions, 5 to physiotherapist-written instructions and 5 to self-written instructions. After 1 week compare their self-reported compliance (on a 5 point scale where 5 = did every exercise daily, 1 = did no exercises at all). The results are as follows:

Subject	Condition 1 Oral	Rank	Subject	Condition 2 Physio.	Rank	Subject	Condition 3 Self	Rank
1	3		1	3		1	4	
2	2		2	3		2	3	
3	2		3	3		3	4	
4	3		4	2		4	3	
5	1		5	3		5	5	

State the H and p values in the format recommended earlier.

2. Jonckheere trend test

This test is used with the same experimental designs as the Kruskal-Wallis, i.e.

— three or more different (unmatched) subject groups are being compared
— the data is ordinal or interval/ratio
— the conditions required for a parametric test cannot be fulfilled (see p. 147 for the design).

However, the one major difference which determines whether you use a Kruskal-Wallis or Jonckheere trend test relates to your hypothesis. If you simply predict that there will be differences between the groups, without specifying which group will perform best or worst then you use the Kruskal-Wallis. However, if you predict a *trend* in your results, e.g.

Group A will do better than Group B who in turn will do better than Group C

then you are predicting a definite direction to your results and you should use the Jonckheere to analyse them.

When calculating the Jonckheere, you end up with a numerical value for S, which you look up in the probability tables associated with the Jonckheere test, to see whether this value represents a significant trend in the results.

It should be stressed here that you *must* have the same numbers of subjects in each group for the Jonckheere. This is not necessary for the Kruskal-Wallis, but it is an essential here.

Example

Therefore, if we look back at the example given on page 159, i.e. that there will be a difference in the strength of muscle contraction in the biceps of stroke patients according to the type of preparation used, we can see that because we only predicted a difference in efficacy without specifying which preparation would be best, we used a Kruskal-Wallis. However, if we restated that hypothesis to predict a specific direction to the results:

H_1 There is a difference in the strength of the biceps muscle contraction in stroke patients according to the type of preparation used, *with 2 minutes' specific warm-up being more effective than 2 minutes' general warm-up which in turn is more effective than 2 minutes' infrared.*

we are predicting a specific directional trend to the results which would require the Jonckheere trend test to analyse them. We would therefore have the following design:

Subject group 1 10 stroke patients	takes part in	*Condition 1* Specific warm-up	Groups are compared on strength of muscle contraction, predicting that Group 1 will do better than Group 2 who, in turn, will do better than Group 3.
Subjects group 2 10 stroke patients	takes part in	*Condition 2* General warm-up	
Subject group 3 10 stroke patients	takes part in	*Condition 3* Infrared	

If we use the previous data, we can see whether or not there was a definite trend in results.

These results are:

Subject	Condition 1 Infrared	Subject	Condition 2 Specific	Subject	Condition 3 General
1	3	1	4	1	2
2	4	2	5	2	3
3	2	3	5	3	3
4	2	4	4	4	4
5	1	5	4	5	1
6	3	6	3	6	3
7	4	7	2	7	2
8	1	8	3	8	1
9	2	9	5	9	3
10	2	10	4	10	3

Calculating the Jonckheere trend test

So, taking the data from the previous example, we first have to set out the conditions such that the condition expected to obtain the *lowest* scores is on the *left*, and the condition expected to obtain the *highest* scores is on the *right*, and the remaining condition in the middle. In other words, the conditions must be ordered from lowest on the left, to highest on the right, with any intermediary conditions ordered accordingly.

So, because we have predicted that the infrared group will do worst, followed by the general warm-up group with the specific warm-up group doing best, we must re-order the above data to put the infrared group on the left, the general warm-up in the middle and the specific warm-up on the right:

Subject	Condition 1 Infrared	Subject	Condition 2 General	Subject	Condition 3 Specific
1	3 (8)	1	2 (9)	1	4
2	4 (3)	2	3 (7)	2	5
3	2 (15)	3	3 (7)	3	5
4	2 (15)	4	4 (3)	4	4
5	1 (18)	5	1 (10)	5	4
6	3 (8)	6	3 (7)	6	3
7	4 (3)	7	2 (9)	7	2
8	1 (18)	8	1 (10)	8	3
9	2 (15)	9	3 (7)	9	5
10	2 (15)	10	3 (7)	10	4
$\bar{x}$	2.4		2.5		3.9

To calculate the Jonckheere:

1. First calculate the mean score for each condition
   (*Condition 1* = 2.4, *Condition 2* = 2.5 and *Condition 3* = 3.9)

2. Starting with the extreme left-hand condition and the first score (i.e. 3) count up all the scores to the *right* of *Condition 1* (i.e. in *Conditions 2 and 3*) which are *larger* than this score. Do *not* count any scores which are the *same*.

Therefore, in *Condition 2*, only Subject 4 with a score of 4 achieved a higher score, while in *Condition 3*, Subjects 1, 2, 3, 4, 5, 9 and 10 all obtained higher scores. This means that in total, 8 scores in *Conditions 2 and 3* are higher than the score of 3. This number is put in brackets by Subject 1, *Condition 1's* score. Do exactly the same for the second score (4) in *Condition 1*. There are *no* scores in *Condition 2* which are larger and *3* scores in *Condition 3* which are larger. Thus the total of 3 is put in brackets by Subject 2, *Condition 1*. Continue in this way for the rest of the scores in *Condition 1*.

Do the same for each score in *Condition 2*, although, of course, you will only be comparing these with *Condition 3* since it is only these scores which are to the *right* of *Condition 2*.

Because *Condition 3* has no scores to the right the procedure terminates with the last subject in *Condition 2*.

2. Before we can calculate *S*, we need two more values — A and B. To find A: Add up *all* scores in brackets to give the value *A*

i.e. $8 + 3 + 15 + 15 + 18 + 8 + 3 + 18 + 15 + 15 + 9 + 7 + 7 + 3 + 10 + 7 + 9 + 10 + 7 + 7$

$\therefore A = 194$

3. In order to find out the maximum value A *could* have been, had *all* the scores in *Conditions 2 and 3* been bigger than those in *Condition 1* and *all* the scores in *Condition 3* been bigger than those in *Condition 2*, find the value B from the formula:

$$B = \frac{C(C - 1) \times n^2}{2}$$

where n = number of Ss in each condition
C = number of conditions
i.e. n = 10
$C = 3$
$B = \dfrac{3(3 - 1) \times 10^2}{2}$
$= 300$

4. Calculate *S* using the following formula:

$S = (2 \times A) - B$
$= (2 \times 194) - 300$
$S = 88$

Looking up the value of S for significance

To look up $S = 88$, turn to Table A2.9 where you will see two tables — the top one for significance levels of $< 5\%$ and the lower one for levels of $<$ 1%. Both are for one-tailed hypotheses because a specific direction to the results must be predicted in order to use the Jonckheere test. Start with the top table first. In order to look up your S value, you need the number of conditions and the number of subjects in each condition (i.e. 3 and 10 respectively). Look across the top row for the appropriate value of n and down the left-hand column for the appropriate value of C. At the inter-section point you will find the figure 88. If our S value is equal to or larger than this figure, then the results are significant at the level stated in the heading of the table. As our S value is *exactly* 88, our results are significant at the < 0.05 or $< 5\%$ level. This means that there is less than a 5% prob-ability that our results are due to random error.

Had our S value been larger than the intersection figure of 88 (say 131), we would move down to the second table which is associated with a prob-ability level of < 0.01 and repeat the process. The intersection figure is 124, which means the result is *larger* than this value and the probability of our results being due to random error is less than 0.01 or 1%.

Interpreting the results

Because our usual cut-off point is 5%, and our results have a probability level of $< 5\%$ the results can be classified as significant and we can reject the null (no relationship) hypothesis. There is less than a 5% chance that random error is responsible for our results. This means that there is a sig-nificant trend in our results with specific warm-up being better than general warm-up which in turn is better than infrared in aiding the strength of muscle contraction. This can be expressed thus:

Using a Jonckheere trend test on the data ($S = 88$, $n = 10$), the results were found to be significant at $< 5\%$ level. This means that there is a significant trend in the effectiveness of different preparation techniques for muscle contraction, with specific warm-ups being more effective than general warm-ups, and infrared being the least effective. The null hypo-thesis can be rejected.

Activity 31 (Answers on page 286)

1. To practise looking up S values, look up the following and state whether or not they are significant and at what level.
   (i) $C = 3$ $n = 6$ $S = 61$ p
   (ii) $C = 5$ $n = 5$ $S = 68$ p
   (iii) $C = 5$ $n = 8$ $S = 151$ p
   (iv) $C = 3$ $n = 10$ $S = 124$ p
   (v) $C = 3$ $n = 7$ $S = 55$ p
   (vi) $C = 4$ $n = 5$ $S = 48$ p
2. Calculate a Jonckheere trend test on the following data:
   H$_1$ There is a difference in the number of appointments kept at an out-patients' clinic according to the social class to which the patients belongs, with social class 3 being better than social class 2, who in turn are better than social class 4.

Method   Randomly select 8 patients belonging to each of the social classes and calculate the percentage of kept appointments. The data are as follows:

Subject	*Condition 1* Social class 3	Subject	*Condition 2* Social class 2	Subject	*Condition 3* Social class 4
1	100	1	100	1	75
2	90	2	100	2	70
3	100	3	80	3	50
4	75	4	75	4	30
5	75	5	60	5	60
6	80	6	80	6	80
7	90	7	50	7	70
8	70	8	50	8	75

Remember! You *must* arrange your data such that the condition expected to have the *lowest* results is on the left, while the condition expected to have the highest results is on the right.

State the values of *A*

B

S

and *p*; express the results in the format given earlier in the section.

NON-PARAMETRIC STATISTICAL TEST FOR USE WITH THREE OR MORE DIFFERENT SUBJECT GROUPS AND NOMINAL DATA

Extended Chi-squared (χ^2) test

As the name implies this test is an extension of the χ^2 test described earlier in the chapter. Like the earlier test it is used

— with different subject groups
— with nominal data (re-read Ch. 5 if you need to refresh your memory on levels of measurement)
— when the remaining conditions required for a parametric test cannot be fulfilled
(see p. 147 for the designs).

However, there is an important point which relates to the Extended χ^2 test. The ordinary χ^2 test only allows you to use *two* groups of subjects which you can allocate to *two* nominal categories.

This means you arrange your data in a 2 × 2 table thus:

Nominal categories

		1	2
Subject groups	1		
	2		

However, the Extended χ^2 allows you to use
a. *two* groups of subjects and *3* (*or more*) nominal categories.
This means you arrange your data in a 2 × 3 table:

Nominal categories

		1	2	3
Subject groups	1			
	2			

b. *three* (*or more*) groups of subjects and 2 nominal categories:
This means you arrange your data in a 3 × 2 table, thus:

Nominal categories

		1	2
Subject groups	1		
	2		
	3		

c. *three* (*or more*) groups of subject and *3* (*or more*) nominal categories.

This means you arrange your data in a 3 × 3 table thus:

		Nominal categories		
		1	2	3
	1			
Subject groups	2			
	3			

So you may wish to ask the opinions of senior II physiotherapists and superintendent physiotherapists (two groups) on the Griffiths Report — 'approve', 'disapprove' and 'don't know' (three nominal categories). This would be a 2 × 3 table. You would need to use the Extended χ^2 test to analyse the results.

(By the way, I recognise that the heading of this sub-section may be confusing, in that it implies the Extended χ^2 can *only* be used with three or more subject groups, whereas it *can* be used with two groups as long as they are being allocated to more than two nominal categories. I apologise for this, but as you can see, a clear, succinct title was difficult to achieve.)

The Extended χ^2 test only tells you whether there are overall *differences* between the groups and not where these differences lie. As a result any hypothesis associated with the Extended χ^2 must be two-tailed, in that it cannot predict a specific direction to the results.

The data you obtained in your experiment are called the *observed* data. The main point of the χ^2 test is to compare your *observed* data with the data you would have *expected* had your results been due to totally random distributions. In other words you are comparing the results obtained from your experimental hypothesis (observed data) with those predicted by your null (no relationship) hypothesis (expected data). Obviously, the greater the discrepancies between the observed and the expected data, the more likely your results are to be significant. *Always* ensure that you have tested sufficient subjects to obtain *expected* frequencies of more than 5. The easiest way to do this is by using *at least* 20 subjects in each group. It does not matter how small your observed frequencies are.

When calculating the Extended χ^2, the value of χ^2 is found and this is then looked up in the probability tables associated with the test to find out whether this value represents significant differences between the observed and expected frequencies.

Example

Suppose in the course of your work you had had to treat a very large number of patients presenting with back pain. Over the years, a pattern seems to emerge, which makes you wonder whether some racial groups are more likely to experience low back pain as opposed to a more generalised back pain. You decide to find out whether your hunch is correct, by selecting three racial groups and assessing whether they had low back pain or general back pain.

Your hypothesis is:

H_1 Asian, Caucasian and West Indian patients differ with respect to the type of back pain they experience (low back pain vs general back pain.

You might then go into two or three back schools and select three racial groups of patients (with at least 20 subjects in each group)

Asian
West Indian
Caucasian

and simply count up how many patients in each group had been referred *either* for low back pain *or* for other forms of back pain (*two* nominal categories). Thus you would have:

Subject group 1
Asian back pain
patients

Subject group 2
West Indian back pain
patients

Subject group 3
Caucasian back pain
patients

Compared for differences in location of back pain (low or general)

There are, then, *three* unrelated groups of subjects (Asian, West Indian and Caucasian), each subject is allocated to one of *two* categories (low back pain/other back pain) and the relative numbers in each category are compared using the Extended χ^2.

Imagine that you have carried out some research to test the hypothesis just quoted and you have obtained the following data:

Asian	— low back pain	9
	other back pain	21
West Indian	— low back pain	22
	other back pain	13
Caucasian	— low back pain	25
	other back pain	28

This data is then set out in the following table:

	Low back pain	Other back pain	Marginal totals of patients
Group 1 Asians	Cell 1 9 E = 14.237	Cell 2 21 E = 15.763	30
Group 2 West Indians	Cell 3 22 E = 16.61	Cell 4 13 E = 18.39	35
Group 3 Caucasians	Cell 5 25 E = 25.153	Cell 6 28 E = 27.848	53
Marginal totals of types of pain	56	62	Grand total (N) 118

(Ensure that the cells are numbered in this way, i.e. from left to right)
Make sure your subject groups are down the left-hand side, and the nominal categories across the top, although the order in each case is irrelevant.

Calculating the extended χ^2 test

So, to calculate the χ^2 test, take the following steps;
1. Add up the numbers in each *row* to give the marginal total for
   a. Asian patients, i.e. $9 + 21 = 30$
   b. West Indian patients, i.e. $22 + 13 = 35$
   c. Caucasian patients, i.e. $25 + 28 = 53$
2. Add up the numbers in each *column* to give the marginal totals for
   a. low back pain, i.e. $9 + 22 + 25 = 56$
   b. other back pain, i.e. $21 + 13 + 28 = 62$
3. Add up *either* the marginal totals for patients
   i.e. $30 + 35 + 53 = 118$
   or the marginal totals for types of pain
   i.e. $56 + 62 = 118$
   to give the Grand Total (N)
   $\therefore N = 118$
4. Calculate the *expected* frequency (E) for each cell by multiplying the two relevant marginal totals together and dividing by N.
   Cell 1, $E = \dfrac{30 \times 56}{118}$

$$= 14.237$$

Cell 2, $E = \dfrac{30 \times 62}{118}$

$$= 15.763$$

Cell 3, $E = \dfrac{35 \times 56}{118}$

$$= 16.61$$

Cell 4, $E = \dfrac{35 \times 62}{118}$

$$= 18.39$$

Cell 5, $E = \dfrac{53 \times 56}{118}$

$$= 25.153$$

Cell 6, $E = \dfrac{53 \times 62}{118}$

$$= 27.848$$

Enter each expected frequency in the lower right-hand corner of the appropriate cell.

5. Calculate the following formula for χ^2

$$\chi^2 = \sum \frac{(O - E)^2}{E}$$

O = observed frequencies for each cell (i.e. your *actual* data)
E = expected frequencies for each cell
Σ = sum or total of all calculations to the right of the sign.

Cell 1 $= \dfrac{(9 - 14.237)^2}{14.237}$

$$= 1.926$$

Cell 2 $= \dfrac{(21 - 15.763)^2}{15.763}$

$$= 1.74$$

Cell 3 $= \dfrac{(22 - 16.61)^2}{16.61}$

$$= 1.75$$

Cell 4 $= \dfrac{(13 - 18.39)^2}{18.39}$

$$= 1.58$$

Cell 5 $= \dfrac{(25 - 25.153)^2}{25.153}$

$$= 0$$

Cell 6 $= \dfrac{(28 - 27.848)^2}{27.848}$

$$= 0$$

6. All these values are added together to give χ^2

$$\chi^2 = \sum \frac{(O - E)^2}{E}$$

i.e. 1.926 + 1.74 + 1.75 + 1.58 + 0 + 0
= 6.996
∴ χ^2 – 6.996

7. To look up the value χ^2 = 6.996, you will also need degrees of freedom (df) value.

i.e. $(r - 1) \times (c - 1)$
where r = number of rows (3)
c = number of columns (2)

$(3 - 1) \times (2 - 1)$
= 2

Looking up the value of χ^2 for significance

Turn to Table A2.1. You will see down the left-hand column, different df values. Find our df = 2 value. To the right of this are 5 numbers, called *critical values* of χ^2:

4.60   5.99   7.82   9.21   13.82

Each critical value is associated with the *p* value at the top of its column, e.g. 9.21 has a *p* value of .01. To be significant at a particular level, our χ^2 value must be *equal* to or *larger* than one of these critical values. (Remember that the Extended χ^2 can only determine whether there are overall differences in the results, so the associated hypothesis must be two-tailed.)

Our χ^2 value of 6.996 is *larger* than 5.99 but smaller than 7.82. This means that our results are not good enough to be significant at 0.02, but they are slightly better than the 0.05 level. Therefore we express this as p < 0.05 (less than 0.05). Had our χ^2 value been 5.99 exactly we would have expressed this as p = 0.05. This means that our χ^2 value is significant at the < 0.05 level or < 5% level. In other words, the chances of our results being due to random error are less than 5%.

Interpreting the results

Our χ^2 value has an associated probability value of < 0.05. This means that there is less than a 5% chance that our results could be accounted for by random error. As the usual cut-off point of 5% or less is used to claim support for the experimental hypothesis and our results have a probability of less than 5%, we can say they are significant. The null hypothesis can be rejected and the experimental hypothesis accepted. This means that there is a significant relationship between racial origin and type of back pain.

This can be expressed in the following way:

Using the Extended χ^2 on the data ($\chi^2 = 6.996$, df $= 2$) the results were found to be significant at $p < 0.05$ for a 2-tailed test. This suggests that racial origin (West Indian, Asian and Caucasian) is significantly associated with type of back pain (low back pain or general back pain).

Activity 32 (Answers on page 287)

1. To practise looking up χ^2 values, look up the following and state whether or not they are significant.
   - (i) $\chi^2 = 3.45$ df $= 2$ p
   - (ii) $\chi^2 = 8.91$ df $= 3$ p
   - (iii) $\chi^2 = 6.77$ df $= 2$ p
   - (iv) $\chi^2 = 9.42$ df $= 4$ p
   - (v) $\chi^2 = 7.95$ df $= 2$ p
2. Calculate an Extended χ^2 on the following data.

You are concerned about the missed appointments at the outpatients' clinic and think it may be to do with the case of getting to clinic by public transport.

Your hypothesis, then, is:

H_1 Keeping an outpatients appointment is related to the ease of access to the hospital, when using public transport.

So you select 25 patients who have a single bus journey with no changes, 30 who have to make one change of·bus and 29 who have to make more than one change of bus. You simply note whether or not they missed their next appointment.

You obtain the following data:

		Attended	Missed
	1 No change of bus	20	5
Subject group	2 One change of bus	17	13
	3 More than one change of bus	15	14

Calculate an Extended χ^2 on this data and state what the χ^2 value is and the p value. Present your results in the format suggested earlier.

10

Parametric tests for different (unrelated) subject designs

The statistical tests described in the last chapter are used to analyse results from unrelated designs, i.e. any design which uses two or more than two groups of different, unmatched subjects. They are also used when the conditions necessary for a parametric test (see Ch. 6) cannot be fulfilled. The tests covered in this chapter are the parametric equivalent to those in the previous chapter, in other words they are used when:

— two or more than two different (unmatched) groups of subjects are used in the research and the results from each are compared for differences.
— when the conditions essential for a parametric test *can* be fulfilled (especially the interval/ratio level of measurement).

Therefore, the sorts of designs involved are:

1. Two different, unmatched subject groups, compared on a task

Subject group 1 $\dfrac{\text{takes part}}{\text{in}}$ *Condition 1*   ⎱
       Results compared for differences
Subject group 2 $\dfrac{\text{takes part}}{\text{in}}$ *Condition 2*   ⎰

or

2. Three or more different, unmatched subject groups, compared on a task

Subject group 1 $\dfrac{\text{takes part}}{\text{in}}$ *Condition 1*

Subject group 2 $\dfrac{\text{takes part}}{\text{in}}$ *Condition 2*   Results compared for differences

Subject group 3 etc. $\dfrac{\text{takes part}}{\text{in}}$ *Condition 3*

Results from experiments using Design 1 (two unmatched groups) are analysed by the *unrelated t test*, while results derived from experiments using Design 2 (three or more unmatched groups) are analysed by the *one way analysis of variance (anova) for unrelated designs*. In addition, the

Scheffé multiple range test can be used in conjunction with the anova for further analysis of the results. This will be explained later in the chapter.

Table 10.1 Parametric tests for different (unrelated) subject designs

Design	Parametric test
1. *Two* groups of different, unmatched subjects, each taking part in one condition. Results from conditions compared for differences.	Unrelated *t* test
2. *Three or more* groups of different, unmatched subjects, each taking part in one condition. Results from conditions compared for differences.	One-way analysis of variance (anova) for unrelated designs and Scheffé multiple range test.

Remember that a parametric test is much more powerful than the non-parametric equivalent, in that if there *are* differences in the results from the different subject groups, the parametric test is more likely to pick them up. This said, there are, however, a number of points you should remember:

1. The parametric test and its non-parametric equivalent do essentially the same job in that they compare results from the subject groups to find out whether any differences between them are significant.
2. In order to use a parametric test you must ensure that you fulfil the necessary conditions. (see pp 88–89).
3. If you are in any doubt as to whether a parametric test should be used, always use the non-parametric equivalent.
4. Parametric tests, although more sensitive, are more difficult to calculate.

PARAMETRIC STATISTICAL TEST FOR USE WITH TWO GROUPS OF DIFFERENT SUBJECTS

Unrelated *t* test

This test is used when the experimental design compares *two different* unmatched groups of subjects participating in different conditions (see Design 1, previous page). It is the *parametric* equivalent of the Mann-Whitney *U* test. This means, principally, that you must have interval/ratio data. Do note that because you don't have *matched* groups of subjects, you do not need to have equal numbers in each group. When calculating the unrelated *t* test, you find the value of *t* which you then look up in the probability tables associated with the *t* test to find out whether the *t* value represents a significant difference between the results from your two groups.

Example

In order to rehabilitate meniscectomy patients more efficiently, you wish to compare two treatments commonly in use in your department — audio-biofeedback and muscle stimulation, to see which one produces greater movement in the knee joint. Your hypothesis, then, is:

H_1 Meniscectomy patient who have lost the idea of movement improve more quickly when treated by audio-biofeedback than by muscle stimulation.

You might select 20 meniscectomy patients, all within 48 hours post-op., and randomly allocate 10 patients to audio-biofeedback and 10 to muscle stimulation. After five treatment sessions, you might compare percentage range of movement for each group. Therefore, you would have the following design:

Group 1
10
Meniscectomy patients —— *Condition 1* Audio-biofeedback

Group 2
10
Meniscectomy patients —— *Condition 2* Muscle stimulation
within 48 hours post-op.

Compare percentage range of movement for each group to see if there are any differences

In other words you are comparing the results of two different groups of subjects — a design and type of measurement which requires an unrelated *t* test.

You obtain the following results:

Subject	Group 1* Audio-biofeedback Scores (X_1)	X_1^2	Subject	Group 2 Muscle stimulation Scores (X_2)	X_2^2
1	40	1600	1	20	400
2	30	900	2	25	625
3	35	1225	3	30	900
4	25	625	4	25	625
5	30	900	5	15	225
6	40	1600	6	40	1600
7	45	2025	7	35	1225
8	35	1225	8	40	1600
9	25	625	9	25	625
10	40	1600	10	30	900
$\Sigma X_1 =$	345	$\Sigma X_1^2 =$ 12325	$\Sigma X_2 =$	285	$\Sigma X_2^2 =$ 8725
$\bar{x}_1 =$	34.5		$\bar{x}_2 =$	28.5	

* It does not matter whether Audio-biofeedback is Condition 1 or 2.

Calculating the unrelated t test

In order to calculate *t*, you should take the following steps (the unrelated *t* test formula looks *very* formidable, but please don't panic! As long as you work through the following stages *systematically*, you shouldn't have too much difficulty).

1. Find the total (Σ) of the scores for each condition:
   Condition 1 = 345
   Condition 2 = 285
2. Find the average score ($\bar{x}$) for each condition:
   i.e. $\bar{x}$ for *Condition 1* = 34.5
   $\bar{x}$ for *Condition 2* = 28.5.
3. Square every individual score and enter the results in the columns headed X_1^2 and X_2^2:
   i.e. Subject 1, Group 1, scored 40, which when squared becomes 1600.
4. Add up the squared scores for each condition separately to give ΣX^2:
   i.e. $\Sigma X_1^2 = 12325$
   $\Sigma X_2^2 = 8725$
5. Take the total for each condition separately, and square it, to give $(\Sigma X)^2$.
   i.e. $(\Sigma X_1)^2 = 345^2$
   $\qquad = 119025$
   $(\Sigma X_2)^2 = 285^2$
   $\qquad = 81225$

   Do make a note of the difference between the symbol
   $\qquad\qquad \Sigma X^2$ which means square each individual score and then add up the squared scores.
   and $\quad (\Sigma X)^2$ which means add up the individual scores for the condition and square the result.
6. Now (take a deep breath!) calculate *t* from the formula:

$$t = \frac{\bar{x}_1 - \bar{x}_2}{\sqrt{\dfrac{\left(\Sigma X_1^2 - \dfrac{(\Sigma X_1)^2}{n_1}\right) + \left(\Sigma X_2^2 - \dfrac{(\Sigma X_2)^2}{n_2}\right)}{(n_1 - 1) + (n_2 - 1)} \left(\dfrac{1}{n_1} + \dfrac{1}{n_2}\right)}}$$

where $\bar{x}_1$ = mean of scores from *Condition 1*
$\qquad\qquad$ 34.5
$\qquad \bar{x}_2$ = mean of scores from *Condition 2*
$\qquad\qquad$ i.e. 28.5
$\qquad \Sigma X_1^2$ = the square of each individual score from *Condition 1*, totalled
$\qquad\qquad$ = 12325
$\qquad \Sigma X_2^2$ = the square of each individual score from *Condition 2*, totalled
$\qquad\qquad$ = 8725

$(\Sigma X_1)^2$ = the total of the individual scores from *Condition 1*, squared

i.e. 345^2

= 119025

$(\Sigma X_2)^2$ = the total of the individual scores from *Condition 2*, squared

i.e. 285^2

= 81225

n_1 = number of Ss in *Condition 1*

= 10

n_2 = number of Ss in *Condition 2*

= 10

If we substitute these values in the formula:

$$t = \frac{34.5 - 28.5}{\sqrt{\frac{\left(12325 - \frac{119025}{10}\right) + \left(8725 - \frac{81225}{10}\right)}{(10-1) + (10-1)} \times \left(\frac{1}{10} + \frac{1}{10}\right)}}$$

$$t = \frac{6}{\sqrt{\frac{422.5 + 602.5}{18} \times \frac{1}{5}}}$$

$$= \frac{6}{\sqrt{56.944 \times 0.2}}$$

$$= \frac{6}{3.375}$$

$$\therefore t = 1.778^*$$

7. Calculate the degrees of freedom from the formula:

$$df = (n_1 - 1) + (n_2 - 1)$$
$$= (10 - 1) + (10 - 1)$$
$$= 18$$

Looking up the value of t for significance

To look up the value $t = 1.778$, with df $= 18$, turn to Table A2.5. Down the left-hand column, you will find values of df. Look down the column until you find df $= 18$. To the right of this, you will see six numbers, called *critical values* of t:

| 1.330 | 1.734 | 2.101 | 2.552 | 2.878 | 3.922 |

*$^*(NB$ It does not matter if your t value is + or − because you ignore the sign anyway.)

Each critical value represents a different level of probability as indicated by the bold type at the top of the table. Therefore, 2.552, for example, is associated with a probability of 0.01 for a one-tailed and 0.02 for a two-tailed test. To be significant at one of these levels, our t value must be *equal* to or *larger* than the associated critical t value in the table.

Our t value is larger than 1.734

but smaller than 2.101

Therefore, we must use the critical t value of 1.734. This value is associated with a probability level of 0.05 (one-tailed) and 0.10 (two-tailed). Because our hypothesis predicted that Audio-biofeedback would be *more* effective than muscle stimulation, we have a one-tailed hypothesis.

But because our t value is *larger* than 1.724 it means that our p value is *even less than* 0.05. Thus our results have an associated probability of $p < 0.05$. This means that the chances of random error accounting for our results are less than 5%.

Had our t value been 1.734 *exactly*, the associated probability level would have *equalled* 0.05. This would be expressed as $p = 0.05$

Interpreting the results

Our t value of 1.778 has an associated probability level of less than 5%, which means that the possibility of random error being responsible for the outcome of our experiment is less than 5 in 100. As the usual cut-off point for claiming support for the experimental hypothesis is 5% we can say that our results are significant. However, before we can definitely claim our hypothesis to have been supported, we must check that the results are in the predicted direction (i.e. audio-biofeedback being more effective than muscle stimulation); sometimes significant results are obtained which are in the opposite direction to the hypothesis and therefore *do not* support it.

Here, if we look at the mean scores for each condition, we can see that the average score for the audio-biofeedback condition is larger (34.5 as opposed to 28.5). Therefore, the experimental hypothesis has been supported. This can be stated in the following way:

Using an unrelated t test on the data ($t = 1.778$, df = 18) the results were found to be significant ($p < 0.05$ for a one-tailed hypothesis). The null hypothesis can therefore be rejected. This means that audio-biofeedback is more effective than muscle stimulation for developing movement in meniscectomy patients.

Activity 33 (Answers on page 287)

1. To practise looking up t values, look up the following and state whether or not they are significant and at what level:
   - (i) $t = 2.149$ df = 10   one-tailed p
   - (ii) $t = 2.596$ df = 16   two-tailed p
   - (iii) $t = 3.055$ df = 12   two-tailed p

(iv) $t = 1.499$ df $= 15$ one-tailed p
(v) $t = 3.204$ df $= 18$ two-tailed p

2. Calculate an unrelated t test on the following data

    H$_1$ Absenteeism is greater among basic grade physiotherapists than among senior IIs

    Method   Randomly select 15 basic grade physios and 12 senior II physios, and count up the number of days each subject was absent during the previous 12 months. The results are as follows:

Condition 1 Basic grade		Condition 2 Senior II	
Subject	Score	Subject	Score
1	18	1	17
2	22	2	12
3	10	3	15
4	14	4	10
5	25	5	19
6	19	6	8
7	17	7	5
8	28	8	14
9	18	9	18
10	14	10	21
11	15	11	20
12	22	12	16
13	23		
14	19		
15	24		

State the t, df and p values, using the format outlined earlier.

PARAMETRIC STATISTICAL TEST FOR USE WITH THREE OR MORE GROUPS OF DIFFERENT SUBJECTS

One-way analysis of variance (anova) for unrelated (different subject) designs

The one-way anova for unrelated designs is the parametric equivalent of the Kruskal-Wallis test, i.e. it is used to compare results from *three or more* conditions, with different, unmatched subject groups in each condition:

Subject group 1	takes part in	*Condition 1*	Results from
Subject group 2	takes part in	*Condition 2*	each condition compared for
Subject group 3 (etc.)	takes part in	*Condition 3*	differences

It is used when the pre-requisite conditions for a parametric test can be fulfilled, i.e.:

— the data is of interval/ratio level

— the data is (more or less) normally distributed
— the variability of scores for each condition is similar
— the subjects are randomly selected from the populations they represent (see Ch. 6).

Despite these conditions, parametric tests can still be used even if the last three conditions are loosely interpreted, as long as the data is appropriate.

The one-way anova is so-called because it analyses results from experiments where only *one* independent variable is manipulated. (All the statistical tests and designs covered in this book relate solely to the manipulation of one IV) More complex designs which manipulate two IVs simultaneously are analysed using a *two-way* anova; those which manipulate three IVs simultaneously require a *three-way* anova. (Refresh your memory by re-reading Chapter 3.) All this is outside the domain of this book.

The anova only tells you whether there are general, non-specified differences in the results from the different conditions — it does not tell you which group is better than the others. (To find this out, once you have calculated your anova, you will need to use the Scheffé test — but more of that later.) Because of this, any hypothesis associated with the anova must, of necessity, be two-tailed.

Essentially, what the one-way unrelated anova does is to tell you whether the differences in scores from each condition are sufficiently large to be classified as significant. But if you look back to the outline design on page 177 you will see that different subject groups are doing different conditions. Therefore, any variation between the scores from the conditions must also reflect the variations between the subject groups.

This source of variation is called *between conditions* variance. However, because different subjects are involved in each condition, it is conceivable that any outcome in the results is due *not* to differences between conditions, but to individual differences amongst the subjects, of inherent variations in personality, ability reactions to the study etc., i.e. the result of *random error*. Thus, this is another source of potential variation in the results and is known as *error variance*.

Obviously, you would wish your results to be the outcome of the different conditions and not random error. Thus, the degree of between-condition variance should be much larger than the error variance. What the one-way unrelated anova does is to tell you whether your results are due to real differences between the experimental conditions or alternatively to random error in the form of individual differences.

Example

An actual example might clarify all this. If we go back to the hypothesis quoted for the unrelated *t* test, i.e. meniscectomy patients who have lost the idea of movement improve more quickly when treated by audio-biofeedback than by muscle stimulation. Suppose we add a further treatment group by ice-packs to this, such that our hypothesis becomes:

H_1 There is a difference in the degree of movement of the knee joint among meniscectomy patients according to whether they have been treated with audio-biofeedback, muscle stimulation or ice-packs.

(note the inevitable change to a two-tailed hypothesis in the latter example). Obviously, what you are predicting here are differences in percentage range of movement between the groups as a result of different treatments. Therefore, you are anticipating a significant degree of between-group variation. However, suppose you picked your subjects badly, such that all the most motivated were accidentally put in the audio-biofeedback group. Almost inevitably, this type of treatment would produce the best results, *not* because of the nature of the treatment, but because of the idiosyncrasies of the subjects. In other words *random error* would account for your results. Obviously, the sort of situation which has all the most motivated subjects inadvertently allocated to one group is very unlikely to occur particularly if you *randomly* allocate your subjects to conditions, but the point is this — your results *could* be due to genuine differences in terms of treatment, *or* to some quirks of your subjects. Obviously, you want your results to be due to the former and what the one-way unrelated anova does is to tell you how probable it is that your results *are* due to the IV and *not* to random error.

Thus, when you calculate the one-way unrelated anova, you have to find out the degree of variation in the scores due to the differences between experimental conditions (between conditions variance) and that due to random error (error variance). This will give you an *F* ratio which you then look up in the probability tables associated with the anova to see if it represents a significant result. Please note, however, that the following formula is *only* appropriate for designs with *equal numbers of subjects* in each group.

Let's suppose, then, that we added this third treatment group to our earlier experiment, such that we were now comparing the degree of movement in three groups of meniscectomy patients following different kinds of treatment — audio-biofeedback, muscle stimulation and ice-packs. Thus we have this sort of design:

Group 1	*Condition 1*	
10 meniscectomy patients —— Audio-biofeedback		
		Compared after
Group 2	*Condition 2*	treatment for
10 meniscectomy patients —— Muscle stimulation		percentage range of movement.
Group 3	*Condition 3*	
10 meniscectomy patients —— Ice-packs		

When we calculate the one-way unrelated anova we need to set out a table for the sources of variance in scores like this:

Source of variance	Sums of squares (SS)	Degrees of freedom (df)	Mean squares (MS)	F ratio
Variation in results due to treatment (*between* conditions)	SS_{bet}	df_{bet}	MS_{bet}	F_{bet}
Variation in results due to random *error*	SS_{error}	df_{error}	MS_{error}	
Total	SS_{tot}	df_{tot}		

So, using the scores from the unrelated t test, together with some new data for the ice-pack group, we have the following scores:

	Condition 1 Audio-biofeedback	*Condition 2* Muscle stimulation	*Condition 3* Ice-packs
1	40	20	25
2	30	25	30
3	35	30	40
4	25	25	35
5	30	15	25
6	40	40	25
7	45	35	20
8	35	40	30
9	25	25	35
10	40	30	35
	$\Sigma T_1 = 345$	$\Sigma T_2 = 285$	$\Sigma T_3 = 300$

Calculating the one-way anova for unrelated designs

To calculate the sums of squares (SS) for each source of variation, take the following steps:

1. Calculate the value ΣT_c^2, which is the sum of the squared total for each condition

$$\therefore T_1^2 = 345^2$$
$$= 119025$$
$$T_2^2 = 285^2$$
$$81225$$
$$T_3^2 = 300^2$$
$$= 90000$$
$$\therefore \Sigma T_c^2 = 119025 + 81225 + 90000$$
$$= 290250$$

2. Find the value of n, which is the number of subjects in each condition
$$\therefore n = 10$$

3. Calculate the value of N, which is the total number of scores
i.e. $10 + 10 + 10$
$$= 30$$

4. Calculate $(\Sigma x)^2$ which is the grand total of all the scores, squared
i.e. $(345 + 285 + 300)^2$
$$= 930^2$$
$$= 864900$$

5. Calculate the value of $\dfrac{(\Sigma x)^2}{N}$ (this value is subtracted from all calculations)
i.e. $\dfrac{(930)^2}{30}$
$$= \frac{864900}{30}$$
$$= 28830$$

6. Thus to calculate the SS_{bet}, use the formula:

$$\frac{\Sigma T_c^2}{n} - \frac{(\Sigma x)^2}{N} = \frac{345^2 + 285^2 + 300^2}{10} - \frac{864900}{30}$$
$$= \frac{119025 + 81225 + 90000 - 28830}{10}$$
$$= 195$$

7. Calculate SS_{tot} from the following formula

$$\frac{\Sigma x^2 - (\Sigma x)^2}{N}$$

where $\Sigma x^2 =$ the square of each individual score, all added together

i.e. $40^2 + 30^2 + 35^2 + 25^2 + 30^2 + 40^2 + 45^2 +$
$35^2 + 25^2 + 40^2 + 20^2 + 25^2 + 30^2 + 25^2 +$
$15^2 + 40^2 + 35^2 + 40^2 + 25^2 + 30^2 + 25^2 +$
$30^2 + 40^2 + 35^2 + 25^2 + 25^2 + 20^2 + 30^2 +$
$35^2 + 35^2$

$$= 30400$$
$$\therefore 30400 - 28830$$
$$= 1570$$

8. Calculate SS_{error} from the formula $SS_{tot} - SS_{bet}$
$$= 1570 - 195$$
$$= 1375$$

9. Calculate the df values
df_{bet} = number of conditions $- 1$
$$= 3 - 1$$

$$= 2$$

$$df_{tot} = N - 1$$
$$= 30 - 1$$
$$= 29$$

$$df_{error} = df_{tot} - df_{bet}$$
$$= 29 - 2$$
$$= 27$$

10. Divide each *SS* value by its own df value to obtain the *MS* value

$$\text{i.e. } MS_{bet} = \frac{SS_{bet}}{df_{bet}}$$
$$= \frac{195}{2}$$
$$= 97.5$$

$$MS_{error} = \frac{SS_{error}}{df_{error}}$$
$$= \frac{1375}{27}$$
$$= 50.926$$

11. Calculate the *F* ratio by using

$$\frac{MS_{bet}}{MS_{error}}$$
$$= \frac{97.5}{50.926}$$
$$= 1.915$$

Insert all these values into the appropriate slots in your anova table (see p. 186).

Source of variance	SS	df	MS	F ratio
Variation due to treatment, i.e. *between* conditions	195	2	97.5	1.915
Variation due to random *error*	1375	27	50.926	
Total	1570	29		

To look the *F* ratio up in Tables A2.6a–d, you also need the df values for each source of variation, i.e. 2 and 27. If you turn to Tables A2.6a–d you will see that they each deal with critical values of *F* for different significance levels:

Table A2.6a = $p < 0.05$
Table A2.6b = $p < 0.025$
Table A2.6c = $p < 0.01$
Table A2.6d = $p < 0.001$

Starting with Table A2.6a ($p < 0.05$) you will see various numbers associated with v_1, which are df_{bet} values across the top, and v_2 values down the left-hand side which are df_{error} values. Therefore, locate your df_{bet} of 2 along the top and the df_{error} of 27 down the left-hand column. Where these two lines intersect you will see the number 3.35. To be significant at the $p < 0.05$ level, our F value has to be *equal* to or *larger* than the given value of 3.35. Since $F = 1.915$ is smaller, we must conclude our results are not significant.

Interpreting the results

Because our F value of 1.915 is smaller than the number observed at the appropriate intersection point on Table A2.6a, we have to conclude that our results are not significant at < 0.05, and that the probability of our results being due to random error is greater than 5%. Since the normal cut-off level for claiming support for the experimental hypothesis is 5% or less, we have to accept the null (no relationship) hypothesis. This means that there is no relationship between type of treatment for meniscectomy patients (audio-biofeedback, muscle stimulation or ice-packs) and percentage movement of the knee joint. This can be expressed as:

Using a one-way anova for unrelated designs ($F = 1.915$, $df_{bet} = 2$, $df_{error} = 27$) the results were not significant (p is greater than 5% for a two-tailed hypothesis). Therefore the null hypothesis must be accepted. This indicates that there is no relationship between type of treatment given to meniscectomy patients (audio-biofeedback, muscle stimulation and ice-packs) and subsequent degree of movement of the knee joint.

Had our F value been larger, say 5.234, it would obviously have been significant on Tables A2.6a's numbers. But could we do any better? Turn to Table A2.6b ($p < 0.025$) and repeat the process. The value at the intersection point using df values of 2 and 27 is 4.24. Our F value is *larger* than this and so is significant at the < 0.025 level. Repeat the process with Table A2.6c ($p < 0.01$). The value at the intersection point is 5.49. Our F ratio is smaller and so is not significant at this level. Therefore, in this case we would conclude that the F value of 5.234 is significant at the $p < 0.025$ level.

Remember that because an anova only tells us whether there are differences and *not* in which direction these difference lie, the p values are for a two-tailed hypothesis. Had you obtained significant results and you wanted to find out which group did significantly better than the others, you would need to use the Scheffé (see next section). However, it must be stressed that you should *only* use the Scheffé if you obtained significant results from your anova.

Activity 34

1. To practise looking up F ratios, look up the following and state whether or not they are significant and at what level:

    (i) df = 3   df = 12 $F = 6.103$ p
   (ii) df = 2   df = 10 $F = 15.76$ p
  (iii) df = 3   df = 15 $F = 4.01$ p
  (iv) df = 3   df = 12 $F = 5.95$ p

2. Calculate a one-way unrelated anova on the following data:

       H_1 Clapping has a differential effect on cystic fibrosis patients of different ages.

  Method Select seven cystic fibrosis patients aged 3–5; seven aged 6–8, and seven aged 9–11. Measure their vital capacity prior to treatment and convert it to a percentage of the normal age-related average. Following 1 month of treatment, measure the vital capacity of each subject in the same way. Compare the *differences* in percentage capacity.

	3–5 years	6–8 years	9–11 years
1	25	15	10
2	35	30	20
3	30	20	20
4	20	15	25
5	20	25	15
6	25	30	10
7	15	15	20

State your F ratio and p value in a format similar to that suggested. Also, present your values in an anova table.

Scheffé multiple range test for use with one-way anovas for unrelated designs

The analysis of variance only tells us whether there are significant differences between the results from each condition. It does *not* tell us which group(s) did better or worse than the others. For example, let's take the hypothetical case given in Activity 34 that clapping is differentially effective with cystic fibrosis patients of different ages. Further, let's imagine that the results were significant. These results only tell us that clapping has more effect on some age groups than others, but it doesn't tell us whether one group benefits significantly more or less. In other words, we can't tell from the results of the anova alone whether there are significant differences between:

3–5-year-olds and 6–8-year-olds

and/or

3–5-year-olds and 9–11-year-olds

and/or

6–8-year-olds and 9–11-year-olds.

If we want to find this out, we must use a Scheffé multiple range test.

    There are three important points which relate to the use of the Scheffé:

— the Scheffé can *only* be used if the results from the anova are significant.
— one formula for the Scheffé has already been presented in conjunction with the one-way anova for *related* samples. The formula for the Scheffé for use with the anova for *unrelated* sample is slightly different although the principles are the same.
— the Scheffé can only be carried out *after* an anova has been performed. It cannot be used independently.

Essentially what the Scheffé does is to compare the mean scores from each condition to see if the difference between them is significant.

When calculating the Scheffé you have to find two values; F is computed first for *each* comparison of means you wish to make. This is then compared with a second value — F^1. If any F is equal to or larger than F^1 then the difference between the two relevant means is significant.

Example

Let's take the example given in Activity 2, i.e. that there is a relationship between the effect of clapping and the age of the cystic fibrosis patient. Suppose you repeated the experiment, with six subjects in each group this time and you obtained the following data:

Subject	Condition 1 3–5 years	Condition 2 6–8 years	Condition 3 9–11 years
1	35	20	10
2	30	25	15
3	33	30	15
4	30	20	20
5	25	25	20
6	25	15	10
Σ	178	135	90
$\bar{x}$	29.667	22.5	15.0

You can perform a one-way anova for unrelated designs on the data. The outcome looks like this:

Source of variance	SS	df	MS	F ratio
Variation due to treatment, i.e. *between* the conditions	645.445	2	322.723	15.088
Variation due to random *error*	320.833	15	21.389	
Total	966.278	17		

$F = 15.088$ is significant at $p < 0.001$.

This means that there are significant differences in before/after vital capacities between the three groups of cystic fibrosis patient. However, in order to find out whether one group does significantly better than another as a result of clapping we need to compare:

1. 3–5-year-olds and 6–8-year-olds
2. 3–5-year-olds and 9–11-year-olds
3. 6–8-year-olds and 9–11-year-olds

using the Scheffé multiple range test.

Calculating the Scheffé multiple range test

1. Calculate the mean score for each group:
   i.e. *Condition 1* 3–5-year-olds   = 29.667 $(\bar{x}_1)$
        Condition 2 6–8-year-olds   = 22.5 $(\bar{x}_2)$
        Condition 3 9–11-year-olds   = 15.0 $(\bar{x}_3)$
2. Find the value of F for the first comparison you wish to make, i.e.
                3–5-years-olds vs 6–8-year-olds
   using the following formula:

$$F = \frac{(\bar{x}_1 - \bar{x}_2)^2}{\dfrac{MS_{error}}{n_1} + \dfrac{MS_{error}}{n_2}}$$

where $\bar{x}_1$ = mean for *Condition 1*
                  = 29.667
      $\bar{x}_2$ = mean for *Condition 2*
                  = 22.5
      MS_{error} = the MS_{error} value from the anova table
                   = 21.389
      n_1 = the number of subjects in *Condition 1*
            = 6
      n_2 = the number of subjects in *Condition 2*
            = 6

Substituting these values:

$$F = \frac{(29.667 - 22.5)^2}{\dfrac{21.389}{6} + \dfrac{21.389}{6}}$$

$$\frac{(7.167)^2}{3.565 + 3.565}$$

$$= \frac{51.366}{7.13}$$

$$= 7.204$$

3. Repeat the calculations for the second comparison, i.e.
                3–5-year-olds vs 9–11-year-olds.
   Substitute the appropriate means and n values.

$$\therefore F = \frac{(\bar{x}_1 - \bar{x}_3)^2}{\dfrac{MS_{error}}{n_1} + \dfrac{MS_{error}}{n_3}}$$

$$= \frac{(29.667 - 15)^2}{\dfrac{21.389}{6} + \dfrac{21.389}{6}}$$

$$= 30.171$$

4. Repeat the calculations for the third comparison, i.e.

6–8-year-olds vs 9–11-year-olds.

Substitute the appropriate means and n values.

$$\therefore F = \frac{(\bar{x}_2 - \bar{x}_3)^2}{\dfrac{MS_{error}}{n_2} + \dfrac{MS_{error}}{n_3}}$$

$$= \frac{(22.5 - 15)^2}{\dfrac{21.389}{6} + \dfrac{21.389}{6}}$$

$$= 7.889$$

5. To calculate F^1, use the df_{bet} and the df_{error} values derived from the anova table (i.e. 2 and 15 respectively). Turn to Table A2.6a: critical values of F at $p < 0.05$. Locate df_{bet} (2) across the top row and df_{error} (15) down the left-hand column. At their intersection point, you will see the figure 3.68.

Find the F^1 from the formula

$$F^1 = (C - 1) \, F^\circ$$

where F° is the figure at the intersection point

          = 3.68

          C is the number of conditions

          = 3

$$F^1 = (3 - 1) \, 3.68$$

$$= 7.36$$

6. Compare each F value derived from the comparison of pairs of means with the F^1 value above. If the F value is equal to or larger than F^1, then the result is significant at $p < 0.05$ (because we used the $p < 0.05$ table to calculate F^1).

If we take our F values:

1. 7.204
2. 30.171
3. 7.889

we can see that only comparison (1) is not significant (3–5-year-olds vs 6–8-year-olds).

This means that the differences between

3–5-year-olds and 9–11-year-olds
6–8-years-olds and 9–11-year-olds

are significant and that there is less than a 5% probability that the results are due to random error.

It is important to point out that to derive F^1 we used the $p < 0.05$ table. The reason for this relates to the extreme stringency of the Scheffé — if we were to derive F^1 from the smaller p value tables, we would rarely get significant results using the Scheffé.

However, should you ever obtain results from the Scheffé which look as though they might be significant at a lower p value, just re-calculate F^1 using Tables A2.6a–d. Here, the F value of 30.71 (comparison 2) above seems to be significant at a smaller probability level. If we recalculate F^1 using Table A2.6d ($p < 0.001$) we get

$$(3 - 1)\ 11.34$$
$$F^1 = 22.68$$

The F value of 30.171 is larger than this and so this comparison (3–5-year-olds vs 9–11-year-olds) is significant at $p < 0.001$.

Interpreting the results

We have obtained the following results:

1. The comparison between the 3–5 and 6–8-year-olds was not significant. This means that any differences between these two groups could be explained by random error. Therefore there is no significant difference in improvement in vital capacity between these groups as a result of clapping.
2. The comparison between the 3–5 and 9–11-year-olds is significant at $p < 0.001$. This means that there is less than a 0.1% chance that the differences between these groups are attributable to random error. Therefore, we can conclude that the 3–5 year group benefits from clapping significantly more than the 9–11 year group (mean scores 29.667 and 15.0 respectively).
3. The comparison between the 6–8 and 9–11-year-olds is significant at $p < 0.05$. Therefore, there is less than a 5% probability that random error could account for the differences between these groups. The 6–8-year-old group benefits significantly more from clapping than does the 9–11-year-old group.

These results might be expressed in the following way:

Having calculated a one-way anova for unrelated designs on the data and obtained significant results ($F = 15.088, p < 0.001$), comparisons of means were performed using the Scheffé multiple range test. The results indicated that (a) there was no significant difference between the 3–5 and 6–8-year-olds ($F = 7.204$); (b) the comparison between the 3–5 and 9–11-year-olds was significant at $p < 0.001$ ($F = 30.171$); (c) the comparison between the 6–8 and 9–11-year-olds was significant at $p < 0.05$ ($F = 7.889$).

Activity 35 (Answers on page 288)

1. Carry out a Scheffé on the following results:

   H$_1$ There is a difference in the 'A'-level standards of students accepted at a school of physiotherapy over the last decade.

   Method   Randomly select 10 students who were accepted for training in 1975, 10 who were accepted in 1980 and 10 who were accepted in 1985. For each student, count up their total 'A'-level points (Grade A = 5 marks, Grade E = 1). Perform a one-way anova for unrelated subject designs on the data. You obtain the following figures:

$F = 6.01; p < 0.01$

df_{bet} $= 2$

df_{error} $= 27$

MS_{error} $= 2.11$

$\bar{x}_1$ (1975 'A'-level results) $= 6.3$

$\bar{x}_2$ (1980 'A'-level results) $= 7.75$

$\bar{x}_3$ (1965 'A'-level results) $= 10.15$

11

Non-parametric and parametric statistical tests for correlational designs

All the tests described in this chapter are for use with *correlational* designs rather than experimental designs. Let's recap on the characteristics of correlational designs.

Firstly, while the experimental design is concerned with finding *differences* between sets of scores, the correlational design looks for the degree of *association* between them. Furthermore, with a correlational design neither of the two variables in the hypothesis is manipulated. Therefore, there is no IV or DV. As a result, a correlational design cannot ascertain which variable is having an effect on the other and thus, no cause and effect can be determined. All that can be concluded is whether or not there is any degree of similarity in the scores for each of the two variables. Although this failure to ascribe cause and effect in correlational designs means that the researcher ends up with less precise information than would be obtained from experimental designs, it should also be pointed out that correlational designs are more acceptable if any ethical considerations are involved, because the researcher is not *manipulating* anything. Therefore, correlational designs are frequently used in medical research.

The way in which this association between sets of scores is assessed involves using the appropriate statistical test, which calculates a correlation coefficient between the sets of scores. This will result in a figure somewhere between -1 and $+1$. The closer the figure is to -1, the stronger the *negative correlation* between the scores. This means that large scores on one variable are associated with small scores on the other. The closer the figure is to $+1$, the stronger the *positive correlation* between the scores. In other words, high scores on one variable are associated with high scores on the other (and by definition, low scores on one variable are associated with low scores on the other.) The closer the correlation coefficient is to 0, the weaker the relationship is between the scores.

To carry out a correlational design, you would *usually* select just *one* group of subjects. These subjects would represent a whole range of scores on one of the variables in the hypothesis. You would then measure each subject on the other variable to find out if there was a relationship between them. For instance, if we take the example, that the greater the number of cigarettes smoked, the greater the incidence of bronchitis, we could select a group of subjects who vary in terms of the number of cigarettes they smoked, i.e. represented a whole range of scores on the smoking variables, e.g.

Subject	No. of cigarettes
1	0
2	15
3	10
4	20
5	30
6	0
7	5
8	25
9	40
10	20

and then collect information on their incidence of bronchitis over the last few years. We would expect that the subject who smoked fewest cigarettes would have the lowest incidence of bronchitis, while the one who smoked most would have the highest incidence, with the other subjects ranging in between accordingly, e.g.

Subject	Cigarettes	Bronchitis
1	0	0
2	15	2
3	10	2
4	20	4
5	30	5
6	0	0
7	5	1
8	25	4
9	40	6
10	20	4

By computing the appropriate statistical test, we could find out whether there is a correlation between these scores. Such a design differs from an experimental design in that although the experimental design would also predict a relationship between smoking and lung disease, it would have to manipulate the smoking variable in order to assess its effects on bronchitis. This would be done by selecting two groups of subjects, smokers and non-smokers, measuring the incidence of bronchitis for each and comparing the results to see if there are *differences* between the groups.

Obviously, whether you use an experimental or a correlational design depends on what you are predicting and the sort of research area you are involved in. If you're still unsure about the differences in assumptions and approach between experimental and correlational designs, re-read Chapter 3. When you have done this, plan out a correlational *and* an experimental design for the following hypothesis:

Activity 36 (Answers on page 288)

1. There is a relationship between age of patient and vital capacity.

Statistical tests for correlational designs

The tests that are covered in this chapter are appropriate for two sorts of correlational design:

1. Those that compare *two* sets of scores to see if there is a correlation between them. In addition, a further test will be provided in this section, which allows you to *predict* scores on one variable, if you know the scores on the other.
2. Those that compare three or more sets of scores to see if there is a correlation between them.

Therefore, the following tests are included in this chapter:

Design	Non-parametric test	Parametric test
One group of subjects; *two* sets of scores compared for the degree of association between them	Spearman rank order correlation coefficient	Pearson product moment correlation coefficient
	If you wish to predict scores on one variable from your knowledge of scores on the other use a Linear Regression Equation	If you wish to predict scores on one variable from your knowledge of scores on the other, use a Linear Regression Equation
One group of subjects; *three or more* sets of scores compared for the degree of association between them	Kendall's coefficient of concordance	—

Both non-parametric and parametric tests are included in this chapter. Each will be outlined separately.

Statistical tests that compare two sets of scores

Within this section, we shall look at two statistical tests, each of which can be used to assess the correlation between *two* sets of scores. In other words, you would typically take a group of subjects who represented a whole range of scores on one variable, and you would compare these with just *one* set of scores on the other variable, to see if they were associated in some way. Like the statistical tests for experimental designs, you can use either a non-parametric test to analyse your results, or, as long as you can fulfil the necessary conditions, (see pp 88–89) a parametric test. The most important of these conditions is the sort of data you have. In order to use a parametric test, you must have interval/ratio data. The tests are:

Statistical tests for correlational designs comparing two sets of scores

Non-parametric test	Parametric test
Spearman rank order correlation coefficient if the data is *at least* ordinal, or interval/ratio	Pearson product movement correlation coefficient if the data is interval/ratio.

NON-PARAMETRIC STATISTICAL TEST FOR CORRELATIONAL DESIGNS WHICH COMPARE TWO SETS OF SCORES

Spearman rank order correlation coefficient test

Example

Let's suppose you were interested in the hypothesis:

H_1 There is a correlation between the length of rest in support splints and the degree of pain experienced by rheumatoid arthritis patients, such that the *longer* the time in splints, the *lower* the degree of pain (i.e. a negative correlation).

You would select a number of patients who had been in support splints for varying periods and assess the intensity of the pain experience (say on a 7 point scale: 7 = intense, 1 = none). You anticipate that if your hypothesis is correct, the patients who had been in splints the longest would have least pain, while the patients who had been in splints the shortest time would have the most pain.

Your results table might look like this:

	Results from the experiment		Calculations from the statistical test			
Subject	*Variable A** *No. of days in splints*	*Variable B* *Pain felt on a 7-point scale*	*Rank A*	*Rank B*	*d* *(A–B)*	*d^2* *$(A-B)^2$*
1	4	5	2	7.5	−5.5	30.25
2	10	3	5	4.5	+0.5	0.25
3	15	1	8	2	+6	36
4	7	3	3	4.5	−1.5	2.25
5	2	6	1	9	−8	64
6	21	1	9	2	+7	49
7	14	1	7	2	+5	25
8	12	4	6	6	0	0
9	8	5	4	7.5	−3.5	12.25
						$\Sigma d^2 = 219$

* It does not matter which is Variable A and which is B.

Because one set of scores (the pain measure) is only *ordinal*, we cannot fulfil the conditions necessary for a parametric test and so the Spearman must be used. It should be remembered that it does not matter at all that one variable is of an interval/ratio type (number of days in splints) and that the other is of an ordinal type, since all this correlational test does is to tell you whether the highest scores on one variable are associated with the highest scores on the other, irrespective of the nature of the scores. Therefore, as long as your data is not nominal, you can compare anything using the Spearman — weight with height, percentage range of movement with pain etc.

When calculating the Spearman you will find a correlation coefficient called r_s or rho, which you then look up in the Probability Tables associated with the Spearman test to see whether this value represents a significant correlation between the two variables.

Calculating the Spearman test

To calculate the Spearman test, take the following steps:

1. Rank order the scores on Variable A, giving the rank of 1 to the smallest score, the rank of 2 to the next smallest and so on. Enter these ranks in the Column 'Rank A'. Repeat the procedure for the scores in variable B and enter the ranks in the column 'Rank B'.

   If some scores are the same, follow the procedure for tied ranks (see pp 112–113). In other words add up the ranks these scores would have had if they had been different and divide this total by the number of scores that are the same. For example, in variable B, the lowest score is 1, but subjects 3, 6 and 7 all had this score. Thus, had these scores been different they would have had the ranks 1, 2 and 3. Therefore, add these ranks up, and divide by 3, (because there are *three* scores of 1)

   i.e. $\dfrac{1 + 2 + 3}{3} = 2$

   Assign the rank of 2 to each score of 1.
2. For each subject take the Rank B score from the Rank A score to give d. Enter these differences in the column entitled 'd (A − B)'.

   i.e. subject 1, Rank A − Rank B = 2 − 7.5
   $$= -5.5$$

3. Square each d to give d^2, and enter this in the appropriate column, entitled 'd^2'
   $$\therefore -5.5^2 = 30.25$$
4. Add up all the d^2 figures to give Σd^2. (Σ means 'sum or total of')
   $$\therefore \Sigma d^2 = 219$$
5. Find r_s from the following formula:

   $$r_s = 1 - \frac{6\Sigma d^2}{N(N^2 - 1)}$$

   Where Σd^2 = the total of all the d^2 values
   i.e. 219
   N = the number of subjects or pairs of scores
   i.e. 9

If we substitute these values then

$$r = 1 - \frac{6 \times 219}{9(81 - 1)}$$

$$= 1 - \frac{1314}{720}$$

$$= 1 - 1.825$$

$$\therefore r_s = -0.825$$

(Do *not* forget to put in the + or − sign in front of the r_s figure, since this indicates a positive or negative correlation respectively.)

Looking up the value of r_s

Turn to Table A2.10. Down the left-hand column you will find values of N, while across the top you will see levels of significance for a one-tailed test and for a two-tailed test. Firstly, find your value of N down the left-hand column. To the right you will see four numbers, called *critical values* of r_s:

0.600   0.683   0.783   0.833

Each of these values is associated with the level of significance indicated at the top of the column, e.g. 0.600 is associated with

0.05 for a one-tailed test.
0.10 for a two-tailed test.

If your r_s value is *equal* to or *larger* than one of these four critical values, then your results are associated with the probability level indicated at the top of the appropriate column.

Our r_s value of − 0.825 (ignore the minus sign for the time being) is larger than 0.783, but smaller than 0.833, so we must select the 0.783 value. Because we have a one-tailed hypothesis (the *longer* the time in splints, the *less* the pain) this means our results are associated with a probability level of 0.01. But because our r_s value is *larger* than the critical value of 0.783, the probability level is even *smaller* than 0.01. In other words the probability of our results being due to random error is *even less* than 0.01 or 1%. This is expressed as:

$p < 0.01$ (or < 1%) (< means 'less than')

Had our r_s value been *equal* to the critical value of 0.783 the associated probability level would be *exactly* 0.01. This would be expressed as:

$p = 0.01$ (or 1%)

Interpreting the results

Our r_s value of − 0.825 is associated with a probability level of less than

1%. This means that the chance of random error accounting for our results is less than 1 in 100. Now, given that the usual cut-off point for claiming results as significant is 5% or less, we can say that the results obtained in this experiment *are* significant. However, before we can claim that our hypothesis has been supported, we must check that the results are in the predicted direction. We have a r_s value of *minus* 0.825. This means that the two variables are negatively correlated; in other words, the *longer* the time in support splints, the *less* the pain. This is exactly what was predicted and so we can safely reject the null hypothesis and accept the experimental hypothesis. This can be expressed in the following way:

> Using a Spearman test on the data ($r_s = -0.825$, $N = 9$) the results were found to be significant ($p < 0.01$ for a one-tailed test). This means that there is a negative correlation between the variables, such that the longer the time spent in support splints, the less the degree of pain experienced. The null hypothesis can therefore be rejected.

Activity 37 (Answers on pages 288–289)

1. To practise looking up r_s values, look up the following and state whether or not they are significant and at what level.

   (i) $r = 0.784$ $N = 10$ one-tailed p
   (ii) $r = 0.812$ $N = 6$ two-tailed p
   (iii) $r = 0.601$ $N = 16$ two-tailed p
   (iv) $r = 0.506$ $N = 12$ two-tailed p
   (v) $r = 0.631$ $N = 18$ one-tailed p

2. Calculate a Spearman on the following data:

   H_1 There is a relationship between the length of lunch-break taken (in minutes) by basic grade physios and their degree of clinical competence (on a 7 point scale, 7 = excellent, 1 = very poor).

   Method   You select a group of 10 basic grade physios, who take varying lunch-break times and assess their clinical competence.

   The data are as follows:

S	Condition A Lunch-break time	Condition B Clinical competence
1	45	4
2	65	3
3	50	5
4	30	5
5	75	2
6	40	6
7	55	5
8	80	2
9	35	6
10	70	3

State your r_s and p values in a format similar to the one outlined earlier.

PARAMETRIC STATISTICAL TEST FOR CORRELATIONAL DESIGNS WHICH COMPARE TWO SETS OF SCORES

Pearson product moment correlation coefficient

As was noted earlier, the Pearson is the parametric equivalent of the Spearman test, in that it is used for correlational designs which compare two sets of data for their degree of association. It may be used when the prerequisite conditions for a parametric test can be fulfilled, in particular interval/ratio data (see pp 88–89).

As long as the data is of an interval/ratio level, it does not matter whether one variable is measured in yards, feet etc. and the other stones, percentages, minutes. The Pearson formula can accommodate different sorts of measurement as long as they are of an interval/ratio level.

Example

Let's suppose you were interested in finding out whether there is a correlation between body weight and range of movement in the hip among osteo-arthritis patients. Your hypothesis is:

H_1 There is a negative correlation between body weight and range of movement of the hip in osteo-arthritis patients (i.e. high body weights are associated with low ranges of movement).

In order to test your hypothesis, you select 10 40–50-year-old female osteo-arthritis patients who represent a range of body weights and each of whom has suffered from the condition for between 36–42 months. You measure the percentage range of movement in their hip joints, and take the average of these scores. The results are as follows:

Results from the experiment			Calculations from the statistical test		
Subject	Variable A Weight in lbs	Variable B Range of movement	$A \times B$	A^2	B^2
1	140	40	5600	19 600	1600
2	128	45	5760	16 384	2025
3	170	25	4250	28 900	625
4	132	40	5280	17 424	1600
5	154	30	4620	23 716	900
6	135	35	4725	18 225	1225
7	143	45	6435	20 449	2025
8	149	50	7450	22 201	2500
9	158	30	4740	24 964	900
10	162	25	4050	26 244	625
Σ	$\Sigma A = 1471$	$\Sigma B = 365$	$\Sigma A \times B = 52\ 910$	$\Sigma A^2 = 218\ 107$	$\Sigma B^2 = 14\ 025$

Calculating the Pearson test

The Pearson formula involves some rather large numbers, as you will see. These may look very offputting initially, but you should be all right as long as you have a calculator.

1. Add up all the scores on variable A to give ΣA
   i.e. $\Sigma A = 1471$
2. Add up all the scores on variable B to give ΣB
   i.e. $\Sigma B = 365$
3. Multiply each subject's variable A score by their variable B score
   i.e. Subject 1 $= 140 \times 40$
   $= 5600$
   Subject 2 $= 128 \times 45$
   $= 5760$
   Enter each result in Column 'A $\times$ B'
4. Add up all the scores in Column A $\times$ B to give $\Sigma A \times B$.
   i.e. $\Sigma A \times B = 52\ 910$
5. Square each subject's variable A score and enter the result in column 'A^2'
   e.g. Subject 1 $= 140^2$
   $= 19\ 600$
6. Square each subject's variable B score and enter the result in column 'B^2'
   e.g. Subject 1 $= 40^2$
   $= 1600$
7. Add up all the scores in column A^2 to give ΣA^2
   i.e. $\Sigma A^2 = 21\ 8107$
8. Add up all the scores in column B^2 to give ΣB^2
   i.e. $\Sigma B^2 = 14\ 025$
9. Find the value of *r* from the following formula:

$$r = \frac{N\ \Sigma A \times B - \Sigma A \times \Sigma B}{\sqrt{[N\ \Sigma A^2 - (\Sigma A)^2]\ [N\ \Sigma B^2 - (\Sigma B)^2]}}$$

Where N = number of subjects, i.e. 10
$\Sigma A \times B$ = the total of the scores in the column
A $\times$ B
$= 52\ 910$
ΣA = the total of the scores in the variable A column
$= 1471$
ΣB = the total of the scores in the variable B column
$= 365$
ΣA^2 = the total of the scores in the A^2 column
$= 218\ 107$
ΣB^2 = the total of the scores in the B^2 column
$= 14\ 025$

$(\Sigma A)^2$ = the total of the scores in the variable A column, *squared*
= 1471^2
= 2 163 841

$(\Sigma B)^2$ = the total of the scores in the variable B column, *squared*
= 365^2
= 133 225

Therefore, if we substitute these values in the formula:

$$r = \frac{(10 \times 52\ 910) - (1471 \times 365)}{\sqrt{[(10 \times 218\ 107) - 2\ 163\ 841]\,[(10 \times 14\ 025) - 133\ 225]}}$$

$$= \frac{529\ 100 - 536\ 915}{\sqrt{[2\ 181\ 070 - 2\ 163\ 841]\,[140\ 250 - 133\ 225]}}$$

$$= \frac{-7815}{\sqrt{17\ 229 \times 7025}}$$

$$= \frac{-7815}{11\ 001.533}$$

$$r = -0.710$$

Looking up the value of r

To find out whether r is significant, you also need a df value, which here is the number of subjects minus, 2, i.e. $N - 2$
= 10 − 2
= 8

Turn to Table A2.11. Down the left-hand column you will see a number of df values. Find our df = 8. You will see five numbers, called *critical values* of r to the right of df = 8:

0.5494   0.6319   0.7155   0.7646   0.8721

Each of these is associated with the level of significance indicated at the top of its column, e.g. 0.5494 is associated with a level of significance for a one-tailed test of 0.05 and for a two-tailed test of 0.10.

To be significant at one of these levels, our r value has to be *equal* to or *larger* than the corresponding critical value. Ignoring the minus sign in front of our r value for the time being, we can see that our r of 0.71 is larger than 0.6319 but smaller than 0.7155. Since we have a one-tailed test, our p value is associated with a probability level of 0.025. However, because our r value is *larger* than the critical value of 0.6319, the associated probability level is *even less than 0.025*.

This is expressed as:

$p < 0.025$

This means that there is less than a 2.5% chance that our results are due to random error. Håd our r value been *the same* as the critical value of 0.6319 the associated probability value would have been *exactly* 0.025. This is expressed as:

$$p = 0.025$$

Interpreting the results

Our r value has an associated probability value of < 0.025, which means that the chance of random error being responsible for the results is less than 2.5 in 100.

Because the standard cut-off point for claiming results to be significant is 5% we can conclude that the results here *are* significant. But before we can definitely state that they support the experimental hypothesis, we must check that the direction of the results was the one predicted. In other words did we obtain the negative correlation between the two variables that we anticipated? Our r value was *minus* 0.71 which means that the results do, in fact, confirm the hypothesis and that there is a negative correlation between body weight and range of movement in the hip joint of osteo-arthritis patients. We can therefore reject the null hypothesis and accept the experimental hypothesis. This can be expressed in the following way:

> Using a Pearson product moment correlation test on the data ($r = -0.71$, df = 8), the results were significant ($p < 0.025$ for a one-tailed test). This means that there is a negative correlation in osteo-arthritis patients between weight and range of movement (the higher the weight, the lower the range of movement). The null hypothesis can therefore be rejected.

Activity 38 (Answers on page 289)

1. To practise looking up r values, look up the following and state whether or not they are significant and at what level.
   (i) $r = 0.632$ df = 6   one-tailed p
   (ii) $r = 0.567$ df = 10   two-tailed p
   (iii) $r = 0.779$ df = 8   one-tailed p
   (iv) $r = 0.612$ df = 12   two-tailed p
   (v) $r = 0.784$ df = 13   two-tailed p
2. Calculate a Pearson on the following data:
   H$_1$ There is a positive correlation between students' marks on their 1st year examination and their averaged continuous assessment mark throughout the year.
   Method   Randomly select 8 first year students to represent a range of examination marks. Average their continuous assessment marks for the year's assignments.

The results are as follows:

Subject	Variable A Examination	Variable B Continuous assessment
1	70	66
2	60	64
3	49	54
4	54	50
5	66	70
6	72	68
7	40	49
8	62	65

State your r and p values in the suggested format.

Non-parametric statistical test that compares three or more sets of scores

Both the Spearman and the Pearson test are used for correlational designs which look for the degree of association between *two* sets of scores *only*, for instance, comparing the theory and practice exam. marks for a group of students to see if they correlate.

However, there will be many occasions when you may want to see if *three* or *more* sets of scores are associated in some way.

For example, you may be involved in chairing an interview panel of four people which is concerned with appointing a new deputy superintendent in the department. There are six candidates for the post. You decide to ask each member of the panel to rank order these candidates in terms of their suitability for the job. Obviously, if there were consensus in terms of choice the decision would be easy, but you know that is unlikely to be the case. So, you will have to analyse the rankings in order to see whether there is *overall* agreement. In other words, you have *one* group of six candidates, who are each ranked by four people. You need to assess the four sets of rankings given to each candidate to see how far the opinion of the panel agree.

Therefore, in this case, rather than having two sets of scores to analyse for correlations, you have *four* sets. Such a design requires a test called the Kendall coefficient of concordance.

Kendall coefficient of concordance

This is a non-parametric test which can only be used when the data is ordinal, i.e. when you have three or more sets of *rank orderings*. This does not, of course, mean that you cannot use this test when you have interval/ratio data; all you would do here is to rank order your data and use the *rank orderings* in the test.

A further point to remember is that this particular formula of the Kendall coefficient of concordance can only be used if the number of people or objects *being* ranked is seven or less. So, for instance, you might ask four therapists to rank order *six* patients in terms of how compliant they are. Thus there are *four* judges (or *sets* of rankings) and *six* objects or people *being* ranked. If you want to design an experiment where *more* than seven objects or people are being ranked, you will need another formula and you are referred to Siegel (1956). However, you should find the formula provided here sufficient for most purposes. One other point to note about this test — both the Spearman and Pearson tests produce a correlation coefficient which may be somewhere between -1 (negative correlation) through 0 (no correlation) to $+1$ (positive correlation) whereas the Kendall coefficient of concordance *only* gives us a value from 0 to $+1$, i.e. an indication of whether there is no correlation at all between the sets of scores (0) or a positive correlation ($+1$). It does *not* give a negative correlation. If we think about this a bit more, the reason for this becomes clear. Where three or more sets of rankings are being compared, they cannot all disagree completely. So in the previous example, Interviewer A may produce a set of rankings which are absolutely the *reverse* of Interviewer B's. If we only had two interviewers, we could analyse this with a Spearman and we would end up with a negative correlation between the scores. But here, if Interviewers A and B disagree so completely, from each other, what about Interviewers C and D? If C also disagrees with A, it means by definition they must agree with B and hence there is some measure of agrement among the rankings. If D disagrees with C, it means they must agree with A, because C disagrees with A. Therefore, all we may conclude from the Kendall coefficient of concordance is whether there is a positive correlation between the scores or whether there is no relationship. Because the Kendall coefficient of concordance only tells us whether or not there is a positive correlation between our results our hypothesis must be one-tailed.

When calculating the Kendall coefficient of concordance, the value of s is found. This is then looked up in the probability table associated with the Kendall coefficient of concordance, to see whether the value of s represents a significant agreement among the rankings.

Example

Let's imagine that resources in your department are limited and you are forced into changing your treatment policy for a group of six cerebral palsied children. Rather than sending them all for hydrotherapy three times a week, you will only be able to send three of them three times per week, with a once-a-week session for the others. Obviously, some children benefit more from this type of treatment and you want to identify them, so that they can maintain their normal programme. So, you decide to ask the three physiotherapists who normally work with these children to rank order them according to who would benefit most from a continuation of this treatment. Therefore, you have *three* judges and *six* people being ranked.

Your H_1, therefore, is

There is significant agreement between the three physiotherapists' judgements of children most likely to benefit from cotinued hydrotherapy.

You ask the physiotherapists to rank all the children, giving a rank of 1 to the child most likely to benefit. The results you obtain are:

	Child					
	1	2	3	4	5	6
Physiotherapist						
1	6	4	2	1	3	5
2	6	2	3	4	1	5
3	6	5	3	1	2	4
Total of ranks for each child	18	11	8	6	6	14

(When calculating the Kendall coefficient of concordance, always set the results out such that the rank orderings from each judge go *across* the page.)

Calculating the Kendall coefficient of concordance

1. For each child add up the total of the ranks assigned, i.e.
   1 = 18
   2 = 11
   3 = 8
   4 = 6
   5 = 6
   6 = 14

   Obviously, if all three physios had been in *perfect* agreement, the child *most* likely to benefit from a continuation of the treatment would have been assigned three ranks of 1 (total 3), the child next most likely to benefit, three ranks of 2 (total 6), etc. right up to the child least likely to benefit who would have had three ranks of 6 (18). On the other hand, had there been no agreement whatever, every child would have ended up with an identical rank total, i.e. every child would have received the same rank from each physiotherapist. Therefore, we would have six tied ranks:

$$\text{Ranks } \frac{1 + 2 + 3 + 4 + 5 + 6}{6} = 3.5$$

   Thus each child would have got three ratings of 3.5 = 10.5. What the formula aims to do is to assess how far the *actual* rankings accord with the rankings for *total* agreement.

2. Add up all the rank totals to give ΣR

i.e. $18 + 11 + 8 + 6 + 6 + 14$

$\Sigma R = 63$

3. Divide ΣR by the number of children being ranked to obtain the average rank ($\bar{x}R$)

i.e. $63 \div 6$

$\therefore \bar{x}R = 10.5$

4. Take each rank total away from the average rank and square the result

i.e. 1. $(10.5 - 18)^2$

$= 56.25$

2. $(10.5 - 11)^2$

$= 0.25$

3. $(10.5 - 8)^2$

$= 6.25$

4. $(10.5 - 6)^2$

$= 20.25$

5. $(10.5 - 6)$

$= 20.25$

6. $(10.5 - 14)^2$

$= 12.25$

5. Add up all these squared differences to give s

i.e. 115.5

6. Find W from the formula:

$$W = \frac{s}{\frac{1}{12}n^2 (N^3 - N)}$$

Where s = the total of all the squared differences between each individual rank total and the average rank

i.e. 115.5

n = the number of judges or *sets* of rankings

i.e. 3

N = the number of people or objects being ranked

i.e. 6

Substituting these values

$$W = \frac{115.5}{\frac{1}{12} 3^2 (6^3 - 6)}$$

$$= \frac{115.5}{\frac{1}{12} 9 \times 210}$$

$$= \frac{115.5}{157.5}$$

$\therefore W = 0.733$

Looking up the value of W for significance
To find out whether these results are significant you need the *s* value, (the total of squared differences between each individual rank total and the average rank) the *n* value (the number of judges or sets of rankings) and *N* (the number of objects or people ranked)

$$s = 115.5$$
$$n = 3$$
$$N = 6$$

Turn to Table A2.12. This gives critical values of *s* associated with particular values of *p*. You will see that two tables are presented, one for *p* values of 0.05, and one for *p* values of 0.01. (Note again that because this test only tells you whether or not there is a *positive* correlation between the scores, these values are associated with one-tailed hypotheses only.) Down the left-hand column you will see values of *n*, while across the top there are values of *N*. Taking the *p* = 0.05 table first, locate your *n* and *N* values and identify the number at the intersection point, i.e. 103.9. To be signifcant at the 0.05 level, our *s* value must be *equal* to or *larger* than 103.9. Our *s* value is larger —- 115.5 — which means that our results are associated with a probability value of 0.05. But are they significant at the 0.01 level? Repeat the process. You will find the figure at the intersection point is 122.8. Our *s* value is smaller than this, so the results are not significant at the 0.01 level. So, we must go back to the first table. Now, because our *s* value is *larger* than the value at the intersection point, it means that the associated probability is *even less* than 0.05. This is expressed as $p < 0.05$.

This means that the probability of random error being responsible for the results is less than 5%. Had our *s* value been *exactly the same* as the number at the intersection point, our results would have been associated with a probability value which *equalled* 0.05. This is stated as $p = 0.05$.

Interpreting the results

Our results have an associated probability value of < 0.05, which means that there is less than a 5% chance that random error could account for the outcome of the experiment. If we use the usual cut-off point of 5% to claim significance, we can state that the results here *are*, in fact, significant, and that we can reject the null hypothesis and accept the experimental hypothesis. This can be stated thus:

Using a Kendall's coefficient of concordance on the data ($s = 115.5$, $W = 0.733, n = 3, N = 6$) the results were found to be significant ($p < 0.05$ for a one-tailed test). This means that there is significant agreement among the physiotherapists as to which cerebral palsied children would benefit most from a continuation of hydrotherapy. The null hypothesis can therefore be rejected.

Should you ever have a situation where there are a number of tied ranks, i.e. where, for instance, a judge has ranked three objects or people equally, this will have the effect of reducing the significance of your results. Try, then, to ensure that your data does not contain too many tied ranks.

One final point. Many students ask why W is calculated, since it is not used to look up the significance of the results. The answer is that W is the correlation coefficient, and the researcher often finds it useful to know this value in order to assess, in absolute terms, the extent of the correlation between results. In other words, the correlation coefficient is often as meaningful as the actual statistical outcome to the experimenter.

Activity 39 (Answers on page 289)

1. To practise looking up s values, look up the following s values and state whether or not they are significant and at what level.
   (i) $s = 96.1$ $n = 4$ $N = 5$ P
   (ii) $s = 117.5$ $n = 5$ $N = 6$ P
   (iii) $s = 124.5$ $n = 3$ $N = 6$ P
   (iv) $s = 103.7$ $n = 6$ $N = 4$ P
   (v) $s = 619.2$ $n = 10$ $N = 7$ p
2. Calculate a Kendall coefficient of concordance on the following data. You are concerned about the variability in measurements of joint movement when using a goniometer. You decide to put this to the test.

   H_1 There is a significant agreement between physiotherapists' measurements of joint movement using a goniometer.

   Method   Five physiotherapists each measure the degrees of knee flexion of four patients using a goniometer. The range of movement recorded is noted.

The results are as follows. (*Remember the data must be rank ordered!*)

	Patient			
	1	2	3	4
Physiotherapist				
1	45	30	50	65
2	45	40	55	70
3	25	30	65	55
4	50	55	30	60
5	60	50	65	80

State your s, W and p values in the format outlined earlier.

Linear Regression (Predicting the Scores on One variable from Knowledge of Scores on the Other)

We have already seen that correlational designs are used when we want to find out whether two variables are associated with each other, that is, whether *high* scores on one variable are related to *high* scores on the other, or alternatively, whether *high* scores on one variable are related to *low* scores on the other. This is a particularly valuable sort of approach in medical research because ethical issues are rarely involved. Correlational designs can tell us whether, for example, blood pressure and reaction to a particular drug are related, or whether traction weights and degree of improvement in back pain are associated, although they cannot say which of the two variables causes an effect on the other; all they tell us is whether or not two variables co-vary together in a related way.

Now, there will be occasions when you might be quite happy to leave your research at this point, having found out whether or not the variables are correlated. For example, in the earlier illustration, you may be content with the knowledge that blood pressure and reaction to drug A are positively correlated, i.e. that the higher the blood pressure, the more adverse the reaction to the drug. This reaction, let's say, induces drowsiness.

However, let's suppose that having completed this research, you are faced with a new patient with a blood pressure reading of $\frac{170}{90}$. Now, from the results of your correlational design, you will know that this person's reaction to drug A is likely to be adverse, since they have high blood pressure. However, let's further suppose that this person drives a public transport vehicle. It is obviously essential to establish whether the degree of drowsiness induced is likely to be a danger to him or his passengers. In other words, it would be extremely useful to you to be able to predict this man's reaction more precisely from your knowledge of his blood pressure. In other words, what you want to be able to do is to predict with some degree of accuracy the scores on one variable from your knowledge of the scores on the other. What you need, therefore, is a formula whereby you can calculate the unknown score. This formula is known as a *regression* formula or equation and is of enormous use in medical research. For example, as long as you know that the two variables are correlated, it can tell you:

— the vital capacity of a man who smokes 55 cigarettes a day.
— the heart rate of someone who regularly jogs 2 miles a day.
— the theory exam performance of a student who achieved 32% in the practical exam.

So, providing you know that two variables are related, you can make predictions about one variable from your knowledge of scores on the other, using a regression formula. The Linear Regression technique can be used in conjunction with either the Pearson or the Spearman test, but the data should be of a type which assumes equal intervals. In other words it should be interval ratio or a point-scale which infers comparable distances between the points (see pp 80–82)

The convention when using regression formulae is to call the variable whose score you are trying to predict, Y, and the variable whose scores you aready know, X. Therefore, in the above example, we are trying to predict the patient's reaction to drug A (Y) from our knowledge of his blood pressure (X).

Now, it is important to reiterate that you can only use a regression equation if the two variables you are interested in have been shown to be correlated. If you look back to page 55 you will see that there are two types of correlation, a positive correlation whereby high scores on one variable are associated with high scores on the other; and a negative correlation whereby high scores on one variable are associated with low scores on the other. If scattergrams are plotted for both of these, we find that a positive correlation is represented by an uphill slope, while a negative correlation is represented by a downhill one. Furthermore, it was pointed out that a perfect one-to-one correlation would produce an absolutely smooth, straight line. However, there are very few things in this world which produce a perfect correlation, but supposing we found that the amount of time a physiotherapist spent with a patient produced a one-to-one correlation with the patient's reported satisfaction with the treatment (on a 9-point scale) such that the longer time spent, the greater the satisfaction. If we plotted the data from this we might end up with the following scattergram:

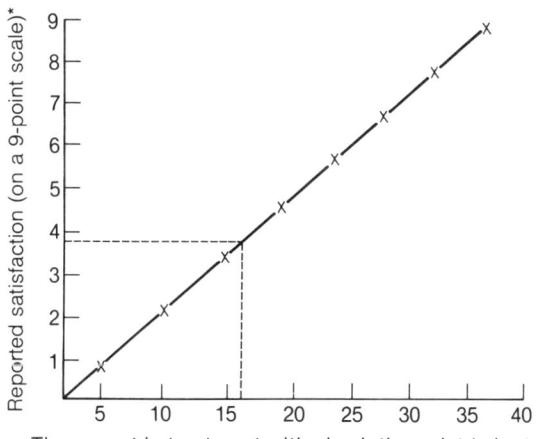

Fig. 32
*For the sake of the example, we shall treat this 9-point scale as though it was Interval data and assume that the distances between each point are equal (see p. 81).

We can draw a perfectly straight line through all the dots and it is this line which is used in your future predictions. For example, you would know from this scattergram that if you were to treat a patient for 17 minutes, the degree of reported satisfaction would be 3.6, because all you would have to do would be to locate the appropriate time along the bottom axis, and trace it vertically up to the sloping line and then move horizontally across to the satisfaction scores (see dotted line above).

You could also predict that if you treated someone for 3 minutes, their satisfaction would be 0.6 — again you simply take the 3 minute time along the bottom axis, trace this up to the slope and then move left from the slope to the satisfaction scores. In other words, from your existing knowledge that these two variables are related, should you ever treat someone for a period of time which has not been incorporated in your previous calculations you can predict how satisfied they will be.

You can see that this sloping line is obviously extremely important if you need to make this sort of prediction and therefore it has to be drawn in. However, while it is easy to draw it in when the correlation is perfect, because all the dots are lined up, it is not as easy when the correlation is imperfect and the dots are more randomly scattered.

However, as has already been pointed out very little in life conforms to a perfect correlation. It would be far more likely in the previous example that the data obtained was:

Patient	Reported satisfaction	Time spent in treatment
1	7	29 mins
2	4	10 mins
3	6	18 mins
4	8	17 mins
5	2	8 mins
6	3	5 mins
7	5	15 mins
8	6	16 mins
9	5	16 mins
10	1	5 mins

Statistical analysis using the Pearson test (see previous section) shows that the data are correlated ($r = 0.836$ $p < 0.005$)

If this data were plotted on a scattergram, we would find the following pattern:

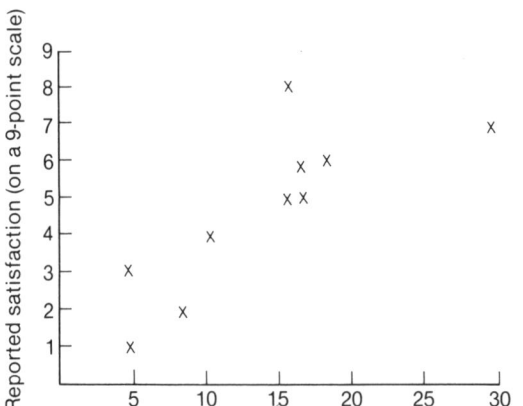

Fig. 33

There is still a general upward slope but it is far from smooth. In this case, if you had to draw a straight line through the dots, so that you could perform the same sort of prediction as before, where would you draw it? You obviously cannot connect all the dots as you would with the perfect correlation and still obtain a straight line so you need to make a decision about where to put the line so that it achieves the 'best fit'. The line of best fit is the straight sloping line which when drawn in, means that every dot is as close as possible to the line, and consequently produces fewest errors when predicting the value of variable Y from knowledge of variable X.

Now, if you look at the last scattergram, you can see that it is almost impossible to draw in the line of best fit by eye, and if you cannot draw in this line, then how can you make predictions? For instance, if you treated someone for 12 minutes, what would this level of satisfaction be? If you only have the scattergram and no line of best fit, you can't answer this question.

What you need, then, is a regression formula such that this line of best fit can be calculated and the prediction made. This equation is

$$Y = bX + a$$

(Note that the regression we are dealing with is called linear regression, because it is concerned with simple linear relationships — see the scattergram.)

where   Y is the variable to be predicted
         X is the known score
         a and b are constants which have to be calculated.

Calculating the Linear Regression Equation

In order to calculate these constants, take the following steps:

1. Calculate the Spearman or Pearson test (whichever is appropriate) on your data to establish whether or not there is a significant correlation. If there *isn't* a significant correlation, don't proceed any further, since you cannot make any predictions from variables which don't correlate.
2. Having established that the data are correlated, make a note of whether the correlation is positive or negative. If you wish, you can plot a scattergram of the data, but it isn't essential.
3. Set out your data in the following format, remembering that Y is the variable to be predicted and X is the variable from which the prediction will be made. Here, we will take the sample data already provided for the last scattergram. So, the X × Y column is: variable score X multiplied by variable score Y
       i.e. for subject 1 : 7 × 29
               = 203
The X^2 column is simply the squared variable X score. Therefore, for subject 1, 29 × 29 = 841.
4. Add each column up to give the totals (Σ) ($\Sigma Y = 47$; $\Sigma X = 139$; $\Sigma X \times Y = 774$; $\Sigma X^2 = 2405$)

Subject	Variable Y _Satisfaction_	Variable X _Treatment time_	X × Y	X^2
1	7	29	203	841
2	4	10	40	100
3	6	18	108	324
4	8	17	136	289
5	2	8	16	64
6	3	5	15	25
7	5	15	75	225
8	6	16	96	256
9	5	16	80	256
10	1	5	5	25
Totals	$\Sigma Y = 47$	$\Sigma X = 139$	$\Sigma X \times Y = 774$	$\Sigma X^2 = 2405$

5. To calculate the constants a and b, first find b from the formula:

$$b = \frac{N \Sigma X \times Y - (\Sigma X)(\Sigma Y)}{N \Sigma X^2 - (\Sigma X)^2}$$

Where N = the total number of Ss
= 10
$\Sigma X \times Y$ = the total of the X × Y column
= 774
ΣX = the total of the variable X column
= 139
ΣY = the total of the variable Y column
= 47
ΣX^2 = the total of the X^2 column
= 2405
$(\Sigma X)^2$ = the total of the variable X column squared
= 139^2
= 19 321

If we substitute our values:

$$\therefore b = \frac{(10 \times 774) - (139 \times 47)}{(10 \times 2405) - 19\ 321}$$

$$= \frac{7740 - 6533}{24\ 050 - 19\ 321}$$

$$= \frac{1207}{4729}$$

$$= 0.255$$

6. Find a from the formula:

$$a = \frac{\Sigma Y}{N} - b\frac{\Sigma X}{N}$$

where N = the total number of Ss
   = 10
ΣY = the total of the variable Y column
   = 47
ΣX = the total of the variable X column
   = 139
b = the result of the earlier calculation
   = 0.255

$$\therefore a = \frac{47 - 0.255 \times 139}{10} \quad \frac{}{10}$$

$$= 4.7 - (0.255 \times 13.9)$$
$$= 4.7 - 3.545$$
$$= 1.155$$

7. We can now substitute the values of a and b into the regression formula
$$Y = b X + a$$
to find any value of Y we require from the known value of X
$\therefore Y = 0.255X + 1.155$

Interpreting the results

Suppose, then, a patient was treated for 22 minutes (variable X) we can predict his level of satisfaction (variable Y) using the calculated values for the regression equation.

$$Y = (0.255 \times 22) + 1.155$$
$$Y = 5.61 + 1.155$$
$$= 6.765$$

Therefore, this patient's predicted level of satisfaction would be 6.765. So it is possible to calculate from any treatment time the associated degree of satisfaction.

Activity 40 (Answers on page 290)

Imagine that the following data were obtained from a correlational study which looked at the relationship between the amount of weight gained during pregnancy and length of labour.

Subject	Weight gain (in lbs)	Length of labour (in hours)
1	17	8.3
2	35	16.2
3	28	12.8
4	21	9.9
5	20	10.0
6	30	15.8
7	24	14.0
8	32	17.5
9	20	11.6
10	26	12.2

(The two variables correlate significantly — $p. < 0.005$)

Three women come in for the last antenatal visit. Their weight gains are: (a) 23 lbs (b) 16 lbs (c) 29 lbs.

What is the estimated length of labour for each woman?

12

Putting the theory into practice

Everything that has been said so far is theory. To carry out a piece of research, you need to put this theory into practice. This section is concerned with providing some practical guidelines to help you set up your research project.

PREPARATION FOR RESEARCH

1. Stating your aims and objectives

It is essential that you clarify in your own mind what the object of your research is to be. All too often students say rather vaguely 'I'd like to do something on back pain/fractures/torticollis' etc. without having any idea what *exactly* they want to investigate. While a general topic area like this is a good starting point, since it defines your area of interest, you will need to develop a more precise idea of what you are trying to find out before you start your research. In some cases, this will involve collecting large amounts of data for a survey. Alternatively, you may wish to test a specific hypothesis at the outset. If this *is* the case, ensure that the hypothesis conforms to the principles outlined on pages 36–37, in that it makes a clear prediction of a relationship between two variables, and *that it is a testable hypothesis*. Some topics in which you are interested may simply not be researchable because the necessary skills, techniques, procedures etc. are not available or ethically acceptable, or because the project would involve major policy changes, which are out of the control of the researcher or would take too long or involve too many people. So do ask yourself whether the hypothesis is testable and feasible.

Furthermore, do define the terms in your hypothesis clearly and un-ambiguously. Using terms like 'safe practice', or 'effective' or 'improvement' are too vague as they stand and you must have a clear idea of what they mean in real terms.

Alternatively, if you are interested in a particular area and simply want to explore it fully without formulating any hypothesis (i.e. some form of survey technique) you will still need to clarify your aims and terms so that you can define the area to be studied precisely.

2. Reviewing the background research

Once you have formulated your hypothesis or defined your survey area, you will have to review all the relevant literature relating to the area you want to investigate. The purposes of this activity are to:

a. acquaint yourself fully with the theoretical background to the topic, so that you have a full understanding of the issue
b. familiarise yourself with all the existing research that has been carried out in the area, firstly to ensure that your own project has not been conducted before, and secondly to provide a context for your experiment. These points are particularly important if you want to write up your research project for publication in a journal.
c. consider the possible methods and techniques of conducting your research.

However, having just said that, one of the purposes of reviewing the research literature is to ensure that your intended study has not been carried out before (i.e. it is an *original* piece of work). There will be occasions when you simply want to replicate someone else's experiment in order to see whether their results apply to your own professional setting. In such a case, the process is slightly different, in that your aim or hypothesis will be identical to that of the study you wish to replicate, and the entire experimental procedure will also be the same. You will still need to acquaint yourself with the background literature so that you are familiar with the theories and related studies, but its purpose is obviously not to ensure the originality of your project.

Do not underestimate the importance of a really thorough search of the literature — there is nothing more infuriating than to carry out a superb (!) piece of research with earth-shattering results, only to be told by a colleague that Bloggs et al performed an identical piece of research a year ago. A full search of the literature will prevent time wastage and disappointment. That having been said, there are a number of practical tips to remember when searching through the literature:

Index Medicus

Use the Index Medicus in your hospital/university library. Index Medicus is, as it suggests, a medical index citing all the medical research which has been published in over 3000 journals. It is produced monthly, and a cumulative volume is issued annually. There are two stages to using Index Medicus. The first stage involves using a volume called MeSH (Medical Subject Headings) which contains all the official subject headings under which articles are classified in Index Medicus itself. It is essential to consult MeSH before proceeding, for two reasons:

1. You could waste a considerable amount of time searching through

Index Medicus for a topic heading which is not officially used. For example, you might be interested in hemicrania. Thus you would look this up in MeSH. You would find the following:

Hemicrania *see* Migraine

This tells you that hemicrania is classified as migraine in Index Medicus and that you should refer to this heading instead.

2. MeSh provides a list of related topics in which you might be interested, e.g.

Mental Health Services
  see related   Halfway Houses
            Hospital Psychiatric Departments
            Hospitals, Psychiatric

Once you have identified all the subject areas which may be relevant to you, move on to Index Medicus itself. The first half of the Index Medicus volume has an alphabetical list of research topics, which is followed by titles of articles published in the area, the author(s) and a reference to the journal where the article was originally published. The second half has an alphabetical list of researchers followed by what they have published and where the article can be located.

Thus, if you just want to find out what has been done on prolapsed intervertebral discs over the last decade, you simply find out the official listing of this topic in MeSH and then look this up in the last 10 issues of Index Medicus and make a note of all the relevant articles, so you can go and read them in the original journal. Alternatively, if you know that Legge is famous for his work on amputations, you would look up Legge in the name section of Index Medicus to find out what he's published recently. You would similarly make a note of where to find the relevant articles and go and read the original. If when reading the article, it *does* appear to be relevant, make a note of it (see next point) and its content. You might also want to look at the list of references at the end of the article to see if there are any important ones which you have missed.

You will find that the journal title is given in abbreviated form. If you're not sure about the abbreviations, you will find a list of all the journals referred to, together with their shortened form in the January issue of Index Medicus.

In addition, many articles, although having English titles, are written in a foreign language. These articles can be identified by the square brackets which enclose the title. The language of the original paper is provided at the end of this, together with information on whether or not an English abstract is available.

If you are just starting a literature search on an area which is fairly new to you, articles which review subject areas are particularly useful, since they provide you with an excellent résumé of the topic as well as a list of useful references. Review papers are listed at the front of each monthly issue of Index Medicus and in the first volume of the annual publication.

A particularly easy way of carrying out your literature search is an on-line computer facility, which many medical libraries run. This is especially valuable if you are interested in a particularly esoteric topic, such as 'Exercise techniques for elderly prostatectomy patients following bladder infections'. However, you do have to pay for this facility (from about £5.00 per search upwards). Information about the availability of this service should be obtained from your library. (It should be noted that there is an International Nursing Index which works according to the same format, but has the drawback of referring to numerous journals which are not available in this country.)

- Do remember — if you are not sure how to use the Index Medicus, ask the librarian.

Physiotherapy CATS

There is also a recently introduced abstract system for physiotherapy journals, running along similar lines, which is called Physiotherapy CATS (Current Awareness Topic Search). This is published monthly, and is divided into two parts. The first part comprises a subject index; under each subject heading is a list of authors who have produced work in the area, the title of their articles and the journal in which it was published. The second part is an author index, similar to that in Index Medicus. All the journals covered are indexed at the back of the volume. There is also a Keyword Index at the back which, like MeSH, gives the official subject classifications which are used in CATS. Each subject classification has some numerical references which relate back to articles quoted in the first part of the volume. So, a very easy way of carrying out a literature search is simply to identify the official classification in the Keyword Index, make a list of all the associated numbers, and then turn to the front of the volume to find out whether the articles referred to by these numbers are relevant to you. However, because CATS has only been very recently introduced, it will only cover the latest articles. Therefore, you may need to search earlier physiotherapy journals by hand.

These Indexes, while an invaluable source of information on the available literature are by no means exhaustive, since there may be research projects on the fringe of conventional medical approaches which are not included or which are thought to be more appropriately classified elsewhere. It is a good idea, therefore, to browse through any professional journals which you think may contain salient articles, as well as textbooks on the topic.

Reference information

Keep a card index of all the references you think are useful. For each relevant reference use one large index card and include, for journal articles:

— the full name of the author
— the date of the journal
— the precise title of the article
— the precise title of the journal where the article appears
— the volume (and part if relevant) of the journal
— the first and last page numbers of the article
— a résumé of the article with all the relevant details.

For chapter references in a book, *where the book has an editor*, include:

— the full name of the author of the chapter
— the date of publication of the book
— the title of the chapter
— the full name of the editor
— the full title of the book
— where the book was published
— the name of the publisher
— a résumé of the chapter, with all the relevant details.

For references to a book which has an author rather than an editor, include:

— the full name of the author
— the date of publication of the book
— the full title of the book
— where the book was published
— the name of the publisher
— a résumé of the relevant information.

You may think this is rather fussy, but I can assure you that a fully detailed card index file is worth its weight in gold. All too often researchers assume (and I have been amongst them) that if they need a particular reference again, they'll know where to find it and so then fail either to make a note of it at all or they make an insufficiently detailed note of it. I can guarantee that by the time you've completed your project and you're ready to write it up, your memory for references will have let you down and you will consequently waste hours in libraries trying to track down a piece of information which you're sure you saw on the top right-hand page of a newish blue book. It really isn't worth the time, frustration and energy so *do* keep a full card index of all relevant references as you go along. And, in addition, if you continue to research a topic, such a fund of references will be used time and again.

3. Deciding how you will carry out the project

Once you have completed a thorough literature review and made sure that your proposed project has not been carried out before, you must then decide on the best method of proceeding with your research. Are you going to conduct a survey, whereby you collect a large quantity of data and then use some form of descriptive statistics to highlight important features of it (Ch. 2)? Or are you going to use a correlational design whereby you measure two (or more) variables to see whether they co-vary in some predicted way (Chs 3, 11)? Or is an experiment more appropriate for the particular project, which will involve manipulating one variable to see what effect it has on the other (Chs 3–6)?

To re-cap on the salient issues involved in each approach:

Survey methods involve collecting a large quantity of data on a particular subject and using descriptive statistics to highlight the important aspects of the data. Surveys can be used for a number of purposes:

— to *describe* the topic area, e.g. how many patients suffer lower leg amputations as a result of circulatory defects, their ages, sex, social class, previous health, occupation, length of time in hospital etc.
— to pinpoint *problem areas*. If, in the above example, you found that 50–60-year-old men who worked in the brewery trade were more likely to have lower leg amputation, this might point the way to further research on any possible causal links.
— to identify *trends*, both past and present. Is there, for instance, an increased tendency towards these lower leg amputations over the last decade? If so, it is conceivable that this trend may continue. If it does, then this might point the way towards developing physiotherapeutic expertise in the area of lower limb amputation and rehabilitation.

Remember, though, that survey techniques are unsuitable for testing specific hypotheses. For this, experimental and correlational designs are needed.

Experimental designs are used to test whether the relationship predicted between the two variables in the hypothesis actually exists. To do this one of the variables must be manipulated and the effects of this on the other variable are then measured. Such an approach has to be carefully designed and controlled, which may involve the researcher in a considerable amount of effort. The results of this approach have to be analysed using statistical tests (see Chs 6–10). However, if the experiment has been carried out properly, the results can provide very useful answers, by identifying causes and effects of certain events. The approach can also establish which of a number of treatment procedures is more effective, which types of patient respond best to particular therapies etc. and so may be especially useful in streamlining and systematising the profession.

However, it does, of course, have its disadvantages. Experiments can be complicated and time-consuming to carry out and they may be entirely unsuitable if any ethical issues are involved. For example, it would be of dubious ethical value to look at the effects of psychoprophylactic relaxation techniques during childbirth on length of labour by comparing a group who had been trained in the technique with a group who had had no preparation for childbirth at all. In such cases, alternative approaches must be considered. One such is the correlational design.

Correlational designs are used to test hypotheses where it would be unethical to manipulate deliberately the independent variable (in the latter case, relaxation techniques) to see what effect it had on the dependent variable (length of labour). In correlational designs, the researcher simply takes a range of measures on each variable to ascertain whether they vary together in an associated way. For example, are high scores on one variable associated with high scores on the other? Or alternatively, are high scores on one variable associated with low scores on the other? Because the technique does not involve any artificial manipulation of patients or treatments, it is easier to carry out than experimental procedures and can more easily be used in naturalistic settings. However, it is for the same reason that cause and effect cannot be established using a correlational design, and therefore cannot provide the same degree of conclusive evidence.

You must decide which of these approaches is most suited to the topic you wish to research.

4. Preparation for the research: Writing a research proposal

Once you have decided on your research topic, carried out a literature review and established which general approach to the project would be most appropriate, it is a good idea to write out a fairly detailed *research proposal*, so that you can plan the structure and specifics of the project. Many people consider a research proposal to be a waste of time unless they are trying to obtain financial support from some organisation, when a proposal is absolutely essential. However, writing up a research proposal has three important functions:

- It helps the researcher to plan the project and to focus attention on all the essential issues, such as aims, methods, analysis and relevance.
- In medical and paramedical research, it is often necessary to check the suitability of a project with ethical and related committees before beginning. For this, a research proposal is vital, since it not only provides the necessary details of the project so that the ethical issues can be fully evaluated, but also demonstrates the researcher's competence, expertise and understanding of the topic area — an important consideration when a patient's health and well-being may be affected.
- On occasions, the research you wish to do will require more time, staff or equipment than is readily available and it may, therefore, be necessary to obtain financial support for your project (see next section). In order to apply for funding you will need to provide the potential sponsors with a fairly detailed research proposal, so that they can assess its value, viability and relevance.

Thus, for these three reasons, it is good practice to prepare a research proposal prior to starting your project. No great detail about writing proposals will be given here, since a lot of the content will be similar to that contained in the next chapter on writing up research for publication. Where this is the case, it will be indicated. Nonetheless, the following information should be included in a proposal in the order given:

a. The title of the research project (see next chapter) which should be clear and succinct.
b. Background theory and the research context for the project (similar to the 'Introduction' in the next chapter).
c. A clear statement of the aim or hypothesis under investigation.
d. The method of conducting the research should be clearly outlined. This is very similar in content to the 'Method' section of an article (see next chapter) and should include a statement of the design of the project, the subjects (type, number etc.) materials, apparatus and actual procedure. In addition, any relevant information about how the public relations aspect will be handled should be included here (i.e. feedback of results to patients, anonymity of the subjects, security of the data, co-operation with other members of the hospital staff etc.)
e. The type of statistical analysis to be used for the results should be included, e.g. if a one-way anova is to be used, say so.
f. The implications and relevance of the study must be highlighted, particularly if the proposal is to go to an ethical committee or a funding body. It is pointless just outlining an experiment without pointing out its direct application and worth to the patients/hospital/staff/funding body etc.
g. The estimated length of time required to carry out each section of the research, as well as the overall time involved, should be included, since this will obviously influence the feasibility and finances of the study. 100 Dupuytren's contracture patients might be difficult to find in a fortnight! Obviously, you cannot be exact in your time predictions because all sorts of unforeseen circumstances will crop up which will delay the completion. Hence, it is better to be pessimistic rather than optimistic on this one.
   If you can draw some sort of chart showing the sequence and timing of the main events, this would be invaluable, both in setting an overall idea of the project and in guiding its execution.
h. If the proposal is to be presented to ethical or funding bodies, then it will be necessary to include details of any personnel (including yourself) who may be involved in the project — either existing personnel or staff recruited specifically for the purpose of the project. There are usually three types of personnel involved in research work:

   — Research supervisor or director. This is the person who takes overall responsibility for the project's execution, directing and rescuing as necessary. If you are the person generating the ideas and submitting

the proposal for consideration by ethical and financial committees, the odds are you will also be the research supervisor.
— Research workers. These people carry out the everyday running of the project, collecting data, administering the treatments etc. They usually have some grounding in research methods or at least receive some training prior to the start of the project. Obviously, careful thought needs to be given to the qualifications and skills required of the research staff.
— Support staff. These are quite often the lynch-pin on which the whole project depends. They include secretarial and clerical staff, computer operators, technicians etc.

In a research proposal, it is a good idea to name the participants involved, together with their qualifications, work and research experience and particular expertise for the job. If you need to recruit anyone specially for the project, you will need to specify the sort of person you want, how long you want them for and what the cost will be. Always remember when you specify the salary range that the appointee will probably only be on a short-term contract and so should be paid slightly more than usual. In addition to the cost of the salary, you will need to add the Employer's National Insurance contributions, superannuation, additional costs and overheads.

Even if you are not applying for any funding it is still a good idea to work out the cost of the project, even if only approximately. You may find that an outcome of limited impact may not justify the expense of new equipment, staff time, computing etc. However, if you are applying for outside money then you should itemise the following costs, overall or per annum, if the project is to last longer than 12 months:

a. salaries, superannuation, N.I. of all staff to be employed on the project
b. any capital outlay on equipment, together with revenue expenditure of any apparatus etc.
c. travel and subsistence costs — if anybody needs to travel to other hospital departments, patients' homes etc., these costs should be incorporated.
d. stationery costs, postage, telephone, typing, computing etc. must be estimated. If you are proposing to handle a large amount of data, your computing costs may be fairly high. It is worthwhile having a preliminary chat with the computing centre you intend to use about estimated costs and the types of statistical analysis available.

Two words of caution, though. Firstly, don't forget to build in some allowance for inflation. Too many promising projects have had to be abandoned before completion simply because the money ran out. And secondly, check out the sort of financial information your potential sponsors require and the format they wish to receive it in before you submit your proposal. A familiar layout and content can go a long way towards getting your proposal seriously considered.

Before taking off on your research, do ensure that not only does it have the approval (if necessary) of the ethical committee, but that it has been discussed and given the go-ahead by all the necessary people. This may involve your superintendent, the relevant consultant, housemen, colleagues etc. It does little for staff relations for a senior colleague to find suddenly that there is a major research programme starting tomorrow, which will involve a total reorganisation of the department. So, do discuss your proposals with all the relevant personnel from the outset.

5. Obtaining financial support

Some research projects can be extremely expensive in both time and money, and you may, therefore, need to apply for financial aid in order to carry out your research. Sources of financial support are many and various and all should be considered as possible sponsors at the outset. Undoubtedly, the easiest avenue through which to apply for (though not necessarily to obtain!) money is your own organisation's research fund. Many hospitals, District or Regional Health Authorities have money available for research, although its existence is not always widely known. However, a relevant research programme carried out on home ground, with direct value to the sponsoring institution or organisation is often a tempting cause and you may find the money forthcoming.

Beyond this immediate channel, there are outside sources, such as the Medical Research Council, pharmaceutical companies, manufacturers of apparatus and the like, all of whom may be suitable targets for your application for money.

In order to decide which of these is likely to be most profitable, it is worth doing some homework. Some agencies obviously favour certain types of research and these inclinations will be indicated by the sort of project they have supported in the past, as well as the nature of their own activities. Obviously, a manufacturer of tractions beds is unlikely to sponsor research into the impact of wearing uniforms versus civvies by physiotherapists, unless the project has some direct impact on their product. Some funding bodies even lay down specific guidelines as to the sort of project they will consider sponsoring.

Once you have decided who to approach, have an informal discussion with them about your ideas, and if they are interested, get the relevant application forms from them, together with any general information they might provide to guide intending applicants. These must be read thoroughly and completed in accordance with any regulations laid down by the organisation.

Some words of advice. The funding bodies are only likely to concern themselves with novel, useful and relevant pieces of work. Projects which are run-of-the-mill or contentious are usually avoided for obvious reasons. Therefore, before applying for money, do think carefully about the nature and implications of your research and how likely it is to fit in with the overall flavour of the sponsor's interest. Also, check the final presentation of your research proposal, ensuring that it is typed, and without errors. Omissions, incorrect spelling and poor syntax will do little to create a favourable impression of your professional competence!

If your proposal is turned down in the end, try to find out why and whether the sponsors would reconsider it if amendments were made. If, on the other hand, it is accepted, then you must keep your sponsor happy. This will involve you in three activities. Firstly, do try to keep within your time and financial budget — funding agencies are rarely pleased with requests for more money or time extensions. Secondly, do send regular progress reports so that they can be satisfied that all is going according to plan (or if it isn't that they are informed about the problem and what you're doing about it). And thirdly, do provide a detailed final report *on time*, with clear conclusions, implications and recommendations. (You might even consider inviting someone from the sponsoring organisation to be on a Steering Committee for the project. In that way, the sponsors can be kept fully informed at all stages.)

All this may seem like a lot of time and effort which perhaps could be better spent on the actual research project itself. Undoubtedly, there are borderline cases where you're not sure whether it really is worth the trouble to make an application for money. This is something only you and the other researchers can decide. However, if you do decide to apply for funding, remember that the sponsors are being asked to invest a lot of money in you and they will obviously want to assure themselves that it will be money well spent.

6. Planning the details of the experiment

If you write a proper research proposal many of the details of the experiment will have been considered and decided upon. Even if you decide against a research proposal, you must make a detailed outline of your plans and ideas for your own benefit, since when you come to write up the research report (probably a considerable time after the completion of the project) you will be surprised at how difficult it is to remember *why* you actually decided on one approach rather than another. So keep detailed notes for yourself as you go along as to the reasons for choosing each methodological or design stage of your research.

At this juncture, too, you should also decide in detail the following points:

— any instructions you will be giving to your subjects during the course of the experiment should be prepared *verbatim*, and typed up.
— prepare sufficient score sheets on which to record the data; if your subjects are to be asked to make written replies during the experiment, ensure that you prepare enough response sheets for them.

— if you are going to randomise the order of presentation of the experimental conditions, or the order of subjects' participation, make sure this is done in advance.

— if you are keeping the subjects anonymous and just assigning them numbers, do keep a record of any relevant details of all the subjects (age, health, sex, experimental condition) on a separate sheet with the appropriate number attached. This is essential if you are to contact them with the results of the experiment.

— prepare for yourself and any other researchers who will be working with you, a worksheet which outlines detailed instructions of what should happen when, and how it should be carried out.

— make sure that you know how to analyse the data, and, if it requires a computer, where and how you can obtain appropriate computing facilities.

— if you are going to use someone else to run the experiment, because you suspect there will be some experimenter bias if you carry it out, then make absolutely sure that the substitute experimenter has only the relevant details (i.e. exactly *how* to carry out the project) and *not* what the predicted outcome will be, otherwise the possibility of experimenter bias will remain.

— if you have to write to people to ask them to participate as subjects, do enclose a stamped, addressed envelope for their reply, and do check just before the start of the project that they are still able and willing to come.

7. Actually carrying out the experiment

A number of points are important here:

a. If you are using any apparatus *do* double-check before you start that it works properly. It is extremely irritating to collect your subject sample from far and wide only to discover when they arrive that the necessary equipment is out of order and they have to go away again. This is the way in which you lose subjects, time, patience and motivation. Also, do make sure you know how to use the equipment properly. While this may seem a ludicrously obvious point to make, it has been known for experimenters to spend a considerable time fiddling about with the apparatus, attempting to find the necessary switches. Trying to convince the subjects of your competence thereafter becomes a major task.

b. Always, always, always run some pilot trials before you begin the experiment proper. Pilot trials simply mean running through the experimental procedure with a few subjects to see whether there are any practical hitches. By doing this, you can establish:

  (i) whether your procedure is appropriate

(ii) whether the tasks you've set your subjects are of the right level; if they're too hard or too easy they can be adjusted.

(iii) whether you've allocated a reasonable amount of time for the tasks

(iv) whether your instructions can be clearly understood by the subjects

(v) whether there are any practical problems in the project.

If you do find any hitches or difficulties at this stage, you can iron them out before beginning the real experiment.

c. Do familiarise yourself totally with the experimental procedure, and what should be done when. It does not inspire the confidence of subjects to see the experimenter scrabbling around for scraps of paper or trying to find out what to do next. So make the running of the experiment as smooth and automatic as possible. The pilot trials should help in this.

d. Treat your subjects well. They are the cornerstone of your experiment and must be looked after. This means keeping them informed (as far as is reasonable) of the purpose of the experiment and of the outcome. Should it ever be necessary to keep your subjects in the dark over the aim of an experiment, because their knowledge of this would bias the results, do debrief them when the experiment is over. Also tell them in advance, if possible, what is required of them and how long it will take. Do *not* do anything which will cause distress or embarassment. People are understandably apprehensive about any form of experimentation, so it is in their, and your, best interest, to try to achieve some rapport with them and an easy, pleasant atmosphere. Lastly, try to minimise the amount of inconvenience subjects experience during the course of the experiment. If they have to make lengthy and expensive journeys at unsociable hours of the day or night, they are unlikely to turn up. Quite simply, try to keep your subjects happy, particularly if they are patients when not only their psychological, but also their physical, well-being may be at stake.

8. Interpreting and disseminating the results of your research

There is no value in simply analysing your results and then forgetting all about them — they must be interpreted fully in terms of their relevance to the profession. What is the *meaning* of the outcome? How does it relate to current physiotherapy practice? What are the implications for policy changes/therapeutic procedures? etc. etc.

However, even this is not enough. If only you are aware of the nature and implications of your results then they are of limited value. The information must be disseminated to other members of the profession. And the easiest way to do this is by writing up the research either as an article for publication in a professional journal, or as a report produced within your department for circulation. While the former method will reach a greater audience, both require the same sort of format and approach. This is given in the next chapter.

13

Writing up the research for publication

Sometimes you will want to carry out a piece of research just for your own satisfaction or to resolve some issue that exists in your own work. However, there will be occasions when your experiment produces such an interesting outcome that you will want to publish it so that the results can be disseminated to other related professionals. Hence you will need to prepare an article for publication in a suitable journal.

A word of caution, though. Good scientific journal-ese comes with practice. Even if you follow the guidelines provided here you will probably not be terribly satisfied with your first attempt at writing up a piece of research. I would recommend that you don't despair and throw it in the bin but instead put the first draft away for a week or two and forget about it. When you re-read it afresh you will probably find a number of points that could be expressed more clearly or succinctly. If you're still not satisfied after doing this, repeat the process. You will soon find that you are able to produce a written style which is suitable for scientific journals at the first attempt.

GENERAL GUIDELINES FOR WRITING UP RESEARCH

1. Always bear in mind that the aims of writing up research for publication are to inform readers of (a) the purpose of your experiment (i.e. the *hypothesis*) (b) the *results* (c) how you came by them (i.e. the *procedure* you adopted for your experiment and (d) what the *implications* of your results are. In other words:

How
Physiotherapists
Resolve
Issues

     involves stating the **H**ypothesis
                 Procedure
                 Results
                 Implications

More details of the basic structure of a report are given in the next section.

2. Always write in the third person not in the first or second person. In other words, use phrases such as 'The subjects were required to ...' rather than 'I asked the subjects to ...'. While this is easy enough when describing the experimental procedure, many students find it more difficult when discussing the implications of their results, tending to write phrases such as

'I think the results can be explained by ...'

The 'I think' would be better replaced by phrases such as 'it is suggested/ posited/hypothesised that the results etc. ...' or 'One possible explanation for the results is .....' or 'The results can be explained by ...' etc. If you have difficulty in writing in the third person, it's often a good idea to take a passage from a book which is written in the first person and simply rewrite it in the third person, for practice.

If all this sounds unnecessarily pedantic, remember that any research should be objective and disinterested. If you start including 'I', 'me', 'my' 'personally' etc the report begins to look highly *subjective* and consequently not very scientific. The use of the third person is a much better style for journal articles (and gives you a greater chance of publication!).

3. Keep your sentences clear and simple and try to convey just one idea per sentence. Remember that your report may well be read by someone unfamiliar with the field, so confronting them with complex grammar or sentences with several adjectival clauses will keep them unfamiliar with it! Clarity of style is easier to attain if you do not assume your reader had any prior knowledge of the specific area. (However, don't fall into the trap of writing as though the reader is a half-wit!) And finally, if you are going to use abbreviations, give their meaning in full at the first mention. For example:
'Twenty patients with leg fractures as a result of Road Traffic Accidents (RTAs) were selected for study.' etc.

4. Do not include any anecdotal evidence in the report, however relevant and interesting it may appear. Science is too formal, theoretical and empirical for personal experience to be introduced.

5. Try to make your article *clear, logical, succinct* and *free of irrelevancies*. Remember always that the purpose of any article is to provide information. Therefore, if someone unfamiliar with your area of research is to understand the article then it is essential that it is clear and logical. Similarly, in order to get the essential points across to the reader, it is important *not* to wrap them up in irrelevant information. The colour of the subject's pyjamas is rarely apposite, although I have seen it included in one student's report!

6. It is important to quote relevant research in your article for a number of reasons. Firstly, it shows the reader that you are familiar with the research area and that you have a number of important facts at your finger tips. Secondly, it adds weight to any argument you produce: if you simply say that 'the administration of lumbar traction restricts vital capacity' the

reader may think 'who says?' On the other hand if you state that 'Bloggs & Smith (1982) found that back pain patients commonly demonstrate restricted vital capacity during lumbar traction,' your argument carries more credibility. (You will note, that I have quoted the surnames of the researchers here, together with the date of their publication on back pain. Some journals specify different formats when quoting research — do check what is required by your intended publisher.) And thirdly, you need to refer to some plausible theory when explaining your results. As you might imagine, theories by identifiable authors carry more weight than anonymous theories which cannot be checked out.

7. There is no one correct way of writing up a report, since each journal tends to have its own format and requirements. It is therefore important to look at the journal's specifications (usually inside the front or back cover) and to read a couple of articles produced in it before starting your own. That having been said, the following sub-headings should provide you with a structure for presenting the essential information from your experiment; you can leave out the sub-headings when a particular journal does not use them.

SPECIFIC GUIDELINES FOR STRUCTURING AN ARTICLE

The title

This should convey succinctly to the reader the essential point of your experiment. It is often easier to construct your title from the relationship predicted in your experimental hypothesis.

For example, if your experimental hypothesis had been: 'Vital capacity is diminished during administration of lumbar traction for back pain', then the predicted relationship would be between lumbar traction and vital capacity. Your title could then be:

> *An investigation into the relationship between lumbar traction and vital capacity in back pain patients.*

To practise producing pithy and clear titles, you could turn back to the hypotheses on pages 42 and 55 construct titles from them.

Abstract or summary

The abstract or summary is a short précis of the experiment. Usually around 10 lines or 100–150 words long, the abstract includes:

— the aim or hypothesis of the experiment
— a brief summary of the experimental procedure
— the results, stating their level of significance
— a brief, general statement of the implications of the results.

Therefore, the abstract for an experiment testing the previous hypothesis might be:

In order to investigate the relationship between lumbar traction and vital capacity in back pain patients **(Aim and hypothesis)** *20 subjects between the ages of 40 and 55 were measured for vital capacity before receiving lumbar traction and again during the receipt of lumbar traction, over a number of treatments.* **(Brief experimental procedure)**
Using the related t test to analyse the data, the results were found to be significant (t = 2.912, p < 0.01). **(Brief results)**
The implications of the findings are discussed with respect to the treatment of patients with reduced vital capacity. **(Implications)**

Obviously, though, you do not include the words in **bold** type and you would continue one section to the next, without starting a new line. (You should also note that all the illustrations are fictitious and *not* derived from any actual research evidence!)

While not all journals require abstracts, they are very useful, not only to the reader who can find out whether the article will be worth reading in full by simply looking at the abstract, but also to the writer who is forced to summarise the critical points of the research in a few lines. This usually focuses the author's mind on the basic structure of the article.

Introduction

The point of the Introduction is to put your experiment into a theoretical context. There are five main topics you should include:

1. It should start off with a general description about the background to the research area. In the above example some reference could be made to any relevant work which has been carried out on vital capacity and back exercises/general traction.
   You might start off by stating something like:

   Over the last few years there has been increasing evidence of links between vital capacity and degree of shrinkage in the vertebral column.

   In other words you have defined the topic area.
2. The next stage is to review the relevant experimental research which relates to this, by briefly quoting appropriate research work. So, you might continue with, for example:

   Brown & Green (1981), in a study of osteo-arthritis patients, found that vital capacity increased following back extension exercises. Similarly, Black & White (1983) compared the vital capacity of cervical spondylosis patients and patients with prolapsed intervertebral discs during traction and found vital capacity was smaller in the latter group than in the former.

3. The third stage involves providing the reader with some theoretical explanation for these findings. Thus:

   One possible explanation for these results comes from the work of Bloggs (1984) who suggested that the effects of the mechanical restriction by the traction harness reduce vital capacity.

4. The next part of the Introduction provides a rationale for your own research, so the previous two stages of the Introduction should be structured in such a way as to highlight the need for your experiment. Most reported research is original; that is to say, the experiment has usually investigated previously unexplored areas. Therefore, the initial part of your Introduction should present any relevant work which has been carried out, and should involve some statement as to where there was a gap in the research. For example, you may find that a particular treatment has not been tried out with a specific patient group, or that a variation on a treatment procedure has not been evaluated. This gap provides you with the rationale for your experiment. Therefore, you might conclude the previous section with:

   However, while numerous studies have looked at the effects of exercise or cervical traction on vital capacity, to date no work has specifically looked at the effects of lumbar *traction on vital capacity during treatment. This provided the focus for the present research.*

5. Finally, you need to state clearly what your experimental hypothesis was i.e.

   The hypothesis under investigation, therefore, was that there is a relationship between vital capacity and lumbar traction in back pain patients.

If you now read just the parts in *italics*, you can get the overall idea of what the Introduction should look like.

Method

The aim of the method section is to tell the reader exactly how the experiment was carried out. It has to be sufficiently clear that you could present your Method section to anybody and they would be able to replicate the experiment exactly without having to ask for clarification on any point. It is usually sub-divided into the following sections (but once again, you should check the journal first).

Design

The independent and dependent variables in your experiment are usually defined here, together with a statement of whether you used a same, matched or different subject design. Furthermore, if you have eliminated any sources of error by counterbalancing, randomising the allocation of subjects to conditions, using a double-blind procedure etc., you should say so in this section. You might state then, for this section,

The independent variable was traction, while the dependent variable was vital capacity. A same subjects design was used, with subjects being measured on vital capacity before and after traction. Each subject's vital capacity was measured by three different physiotherapists on nine separate occasions, in order to eliminate any bias in procedure.

Subjects

You should describe your subjects succinctly, giving all the *relevant* details, e.g. age, sex, medical condition, mean length of time ill, previous treatment, occupation and *how* they were selected. If you just asked the first 20 patients who required treatment for back pain, say so. However, it *is* important to specify whether they volunteered, were press-ganged, paid etc., since it makes a difference to the way in which they react in experiments. Therefore, in the above example, the Subject section might read:

Twenty subjects, 10 male and 10 female, were randomly selected from a back pain clinic. All were aged between 40 and 55; they had been experiencing back pain for at least 6 months and all had been diagnosed as having non-specific back problems. There were no smokers among the subject sample. None of the subjects had received any previous treatment for their complaint and all took part in the experiment on a voluntary basis.

Apparatus

Any apparatus used should be referred to in sufficient detail so that anyone wanting to replicate your experiment can obtain the same equipment. Thus, manufacturer's name, make and type of apparatus, plus a brief description of its capacities should be included. If the equipment has been made specially for you, it should be described in detail and should be accompanied by a diagram showing its main features.

In the above example, then, the Apparatus section might be:

Two pieces of apparatus were used in the experiment. The first was an Akron traction-bed and the second piece of equipment was an electrical spirometer used for measuring vital capacity (Vitalograph).

Materials

Any non-mechanical equipment used should be included in this section, e.g. score sheets, record cards, etc. Here, the section would read something like:

The materials used in the current experiment included patient record

cards to keep records of the treatment and graphs from which vital capacity could be calculated.

Procedure

This sub-section of the method is very important and should include a detailed description of what you did when you actually carried out the experiment. It should be clear, and logical and should provide the reader with something akin to the method part of a recipe, i.e. a step-by-step account of what was done in the appropriate order. Remember that although this part, like the rest of the report, should be relevant and succinct, it should also be sufficiently detailed that anyone who reads the procedure could go away and replicate what you did *to the letter*. The word 'relevant' is important as well — you should only include those details which might have some influence on the outcome of the experiment. For example, the height of a chair a patient sat in to carry out the experiment would *not* be relevant unless you were carrying out research into an area which related to ergonomics or the ability to get in and out of chairs. It is not always easy at first to include just the right amount of detail, but it is a skill which develops over time.

Details which should be included here are things like order of presentation of tasks, and standardised instructions to the subject (which should be reproduced verbatim), how the dependent variable was measured and at what time intervals, number of treatment sessions etc. Therefore, the Procedure section here might be:

> *Each subject's vital capacity was measured in the standard way prior to beginning treatment using the spirometer. The results were noted on the appropriate graph. Each patient then received 15 minutes traction three times a week for 3 weeks (9 treatment sessions in total). Constant traction was given for a period of 15 minutes and was identical for every subject. During the last 5 minutes of every treatment session, vital capacity was measured. Pounds weight on the traction bed were increased in relation to body weight in the usual way. The treatment sessions all took place during the morning and were carried out by one of three senior physiotherapists. The subjects were randomly assigned to therapists in a pre-arranged order, such that every patient was treated three times by each therapist. At the end of the 3 weeks, the 9 vital capacity socres for each patient were averaged.*

Results

The actual scores derived from your experiment do not need to be presented in this section, but may be included in an Appendix. However, it is necessary to include the mean scores for each group or condition. If you present a graph, ensure that it conforms to the guidelines outlined on page 13. Perhaps the most important part of this section, though, are the results of the statistical analysis performed on the scores. While it is unnecessary to include the workings-out you do need to say

1. what statistical test you used
2. what the result was
3. what the level of significance was
4. (a point many people forget) a brief statement of what these results actually *mean*. It is insufficient to just say 'The results are significant at the 0.01 level.' You must *interpret* this for the reader.

So, in the above example, the Results section might be (the numbered points refer to the list above).

> *The mean pre-test score for the subjects was 4.21 litres, while the mean vital capacity score during treatment was 3.13 litres. The results were analysed using the related t-test* (point 1) *and were found to be significant* ($t = 2.912$ (point 2) $p < 0.01$ (point 3)). *These results suggest that there is a significant decrease in vital capacity during traction* (point 4).

Discussion

1. This section starts off with a re-statement of the outcome of your statistical analysis (usually a variant on the last sentence in the Results section), and may add a comment as to whether or not they support the experimental hypothesis. For example:

> *The results of the present experiment indicate that the vital capacity of the patients diminished significantly during traction, thereby supporting the experimental hypothesis.*

2. You should then go on to make some statement about how your results fit in with the findings from other related research. This can incorporate studies which produced contradictory as well as corroborative findings, as long as you provide some plausible explanation for the discrepancy. Here, then you might say:

> *These results accord with those of Brown & Green (ibid), Black & White (ibid) as well as those of Wodge (1983). Wodge found in a study of patients wearing lumbar surgical supports that vital capacity was reduced by 20% due to limitations of diaphragmatic movement. However, work by Jones & Smith (1982) provided contradictory findings. Their results indicated that traction had a negligible effect on vital capacity. However, all the subjects in their sample were smokers and it is conceivable that the existing limitations in vital capacity as a result of smoking minimised the effect of the traction.*

3. You must produce a cogent theoretical explanation for your results and also some comment about their practical implications. For instance

The results of the present experiment can be explained by Bloggs' Mechanical Restriction Theory (ibid). However, the work of Barnes & Bridges (1979) is also relevant. They suggest that when the thoracic cavity is elongated, even marginally, then the lung capacity is restricted. Given that lumbar traction alters the length of the spinal column, it is conceivable that there is a consequent elongation of the thoracic cavity, thereby accounting for the present results.

Furthermore, Gold & Silver (1981) have convincingly demonstrated that any fear-inducing treatment procedure such as that engendered by large mechanical apparatus, causes shallow respiration and a consequent reduction in vital capacity. Taken together these two theories could account for the present results. These findings, however, have important implications for the treatment of back pain patients who also suffer chronic respiratory conditions in which the vital capacity is already low. In such cases, alternate therapeutic procedures should be considered.

4. Next you should include any additional analysis which you carried out and which produced some interesting results, together with some comment on these (ideally its theoretical and practical relevance). For example, you might compare male vs female subjects; older vs. younger subjects; social class or occupational groups etc. In the present example:

Further analysis of the results suggested that the vital capacity differences were greater for men than for women ($t = 2.103$ $p < 0.05$). This finding may be interpreted in terms of the generally larger physique of males, thus accounting for the relatively greater difference in vital capacity.

5. You should then acknowledge any limitations of your experiment — design flaws, unforeseen practical problems that you encountered (e.g. patients not turning up, apparatus breaking down etc.), variables which you failed to control for etc. While this may look as though it is condemning your experiment to the waste bin, it isn't — as long as there are no major methodological flaws which would totally vitiate your results. Most research (especially applied research like physiotherapy) will have some minor faults since the perfect experiment is all but a fantasy. However, if you acknowledge the problems and recommend ways of overcoming them were the experiment to be repeated in future, then your work will not be dismissed as nonsense. The researcher who thinks his/her study is perfect is the one who is more likely to be rejected. For example:

The experiment highlighted a procedural flaw, in that traction weights were not identical, but related to body weight instead. While this may have only limited impact on the results since a same subject design was used, it might have been better to use patients with similar body weights and consequent standardised traction weights.

6. Finally, if your study throws up any ideas for future research, say so. Here you might suggest:

While the study has demonstrated that vital capacity diminishes during traction, it would be interesting to ascertain whether this is a continuous process or whether there is a point in the treatment when there is a sudden reduction. In addition, the permanency of the reduced capacity needs investigating. These areas could form the basis of a future research project.

References

Every researcher you have quoted in your report must be included in the reference section in order that the reader can follow up ideas and theories in the area by going back to the original article or book. Usually, all the names are quoted in alphabetical order and you *must* give the full reference. While many journals have their own formats (which you should check first), there are standard ways of presenting references for books and journal articles. For books, the author's surname is quoted first followed by initials, date of publication, title of the book (underlined), where it was published and by whom. Therefore, the reference would look like:

> Bloggs A.B. (1984) Mechanical Restriction Theory. Oxford: Oxford University Press.

However, you *must* check the journal's requirements first, because if the above reference was listed in a book published by Churchill Livingstone, it would appear as follows:

> Bloggs A B 1984 Mechanical restriction theory. Oxford University Press, Oxford

For journal articles, the format is similar — surname, initials, date of article, title of article, title of journal (underlined), volume of journal and first and last page numbers of the article. Therefore, a journal article would be:

> Black, C. & White R. (1983) A comparison of the vital capacities of cervical spondylosis and prolapsed intervertebral disc patients. Therapeutic Medicine, 14, 15–22.

In the example quoted throughout, all the cited research would have to be referenced in alphabetical order, using the correct format. You would therefore have:

Barnes, M. & Bridges, P. (1979) etc.
Black, C. & White, R. (1983) etc.
Bloggs, A.B.(1984) etc.
Brown, D. & Green, F.A. (1981) etc.
Gold, E. & Silver, S. (1981) etc.
Wodge, A. (1983) etc.

If you go back and read just the sections in italics you should get an idea about the style and format of a journal article, although I would stress again that prior to writing your research up, you should select a journal which specialised in your research area and check the details of presentation it requires.

And finally, just a few tips when submitting articles for publication:

- Do not submit the article to more than one journal at a time. If the journal of your choice turns it down, *then* send it off to another one, but never submit simultaneously. (And always keep a copy!)
- If you carried out the research with colleagues, then it may be appropriate to include their names as authors. Where there is multiple authorship of an article, the person quoted first is usually assumed either to be the most senior contributor (in terms of professional status) or alternatively to have carried out the bulk of the work. However, there is no fixed precedent for the order of names, and trouble frequently arises when the most senior author has done least work but still wants to take first place. So, sort out the issue in advance.
- Throughout the course of any research project many individuals will have helped either by sponsoring the research or helping with any computing. Those people who have made significant contributions should be acknowledged at the end of the article.

I hope that when reading this book you have not concluded that research is a chore, and consequently abandoned any ambitions you had. Of course, if it is to be done properly, then any project will involve considerable time and effort, but there is *enormous* satisfaction to be gained when you come up with interesting results or see your name in print. I do hope you will persevere, and that this text, while not necessarily firing you with enthusiasm, might, at least, guide you in your pursuits.

Appendix 1

Basic mathematical principles

BRACKETS

You will not always meet with straightforward calculations in statistical tests. Many of them have quite complex formulae and it is essential to know which part of the formula should be computed first. One way of indicating which part should be dealt with first is by using *brackets*. Any figures or formulae contained in brackets should be calculated before anything else, or else you will get quite incorrect results. This can be illustrated by the following examples:

$$114 - (15 + 23)$$
$$= 114 - 38$$
$$= 76$$

as opposed to:

$$(114 - 15) + 23$$
$$= 99 + 23$$
$$= 122$$

Brackets can change your answer quite dramatically. Therefore, the first principle you must remember when calculating any statistical tests is:

all calculations contained in brackets must be carried out first.

However, not all formulae are as convenient as this. Some have brackets within brackets, e.g.:

$$14 + [(15 \times 3) - 12]$$

In these cases, you must calculate the formula in the innermost brackets first, then go on to the formula in the next set of brackets and so on. Therefore, the above formula becomes:

$$14 + [45 - 12]$$
$$= 14 + 33$$
$$= 47$$

So, always calculate the formula in the innermost set of brackets first and then work outwards.

ADDITION, SUBTRACTION, MULTIPLICATION AND DIVISION

Although any formula in brackets must always be calculated first, not all formulae have brackets.

Sometimes you will come across something like this:

12 + 19 − 7 − 4 + 8

In such cases *where you have a mixture of just additions and subtraction and no brackets*, you simply start calculating from the left-hand side and work systematically across to the right. The importance of this principle can be illustrated by the following example:

72 − 34 + 9

If you work systematically from left to right, the answer is 47. If, however, you do the addition first, the answer is 29 — quite different and quite incorrect. So the next principle to remember is:

When you have a row of additions and subtractions only and no brackets, start the calculations at the left-hand side and work systematically across to the right.

Similarly, there will be occasions when you have a row of additions *only*, e.g. 19 + 17 + 9
subtractions *only*, e.g. 28 − 4 − 16
divisions *only*, e.g. 45 ÷ 3 ÷ 5
multiplications *only*, e.g. 7 × 8 × 14
or a *mixture of multiplications and divisions*, e.g. 12 × 8 ÷ 4

While it doesn't matter too much in which order these are carried out, it is easier and less confusing if you stick to the left-to-right rule.

However, quite often you will come across mixtures of addition and/or subtraction with multiplication and/or division, e.g.:

a. 71 + 9 ÷ 18

or

b. 117 − 6 × 10

In these cases you *must* do the multiplication or division first, followed by the additions or subtractions. The reason for doing this can be illustrated by the above examples. If they are calculated correctly, the answer to (a) is 71.5 and to (b) 57. If, however, you apply the left to right rule here, you end up with 4.44 and 1110 respectively. So the next rule of basic maths is that *multiplying and dividing are carried out before adding and subtracting*.

To recap on what has been outlined so far:

• First, carry out the calculations in brackets.

If there are brackets within brackets, do the calculations in the inside brackets first.

- Second, if there are no brackets, do the multiplications and divisions first.
- Third, if there are no multiplications and divisions, just work from left to right.

Just one final point — sometimes you will see something like 9 (12 − 2). This means 9 × (12 − 2), except that the multiplication sign between the 9 and the bracket is *assumed*.

POSITIVE AND NEGATIVE NUMBERS

It's easy to get confused over positive and negative numbers. While 40 − 20 is simple to work out, 20 − 40 starts to cause confusion. Perhaps the easiest way to overcome the problems of plus and minus numbers is to think of the left-hand figure as your 'bank' of money in a Monopoly® game. Obviously, you can *add* to your bank or you can *take away* from your bank, but both transactions will alter the resulting amount of money you have to play with. Suppose you started with £200 but then landed on your competitor's Mayfair property, which meant you owed them £300. You have, then £200 − £300. This means that you are £100 in the red, in other words you have − £100. Suppose now that another player landed on your Park Lane property which meant you could receive £200. Because you're already in debt to the tune of £100, half the money you're owed must go towards putting your debt right, which means that you're £100 in credit. In other words you have:

£100 + £200 = £100

However, it's often more expensive than this in Monopoly®. Suppose that while you are £100 in debt, you land on the Strand and owe a further £50. This means you have one debt of £100 (− £100) *plus* another debt of £50 (− £50). This can be expressed as:

(− £100) + (− £50) = − £150

There are, of course, many occasions when you will be either multiplying or dividing plus and minus numbers, e.g.

(+5) × (− 10) or (− 80) ÷ (+8)

Multiplying or dividing a mixture of plus and minus numbers *always* gives a minus answer. So in the examples above, the answers are − 50 and − 10 respectively. Multiplying or dividing positive numbers *only*, always results in positive answers, but multiplying or dividing minus numbers *only also* produces a positive number. If you think about this in terms of double negatives in speech, 'I didn't do nothing' actually means 'I did something.' Similarly, double negatives in maths also mean a positive.

We can state some further mathematical principles now:

1. *Adding* two negative numbers results in a negative answer,
   e.g. $(-20) + (-10) = -30$.
2. *Adding* one plus number to a minus number is the same as taking
   the minus number from the plus number,
   e.g. $-24 + 6 = -18$
   $+6 - 24 = -18$
3. *Multiplying* two positive numbers always results in a positive answer.
4. *Multiplying* one positive number by one negative number always
   results in a negative answer.
5. *Multiplying* two negative numbers always results in a positive answer.
6. *Dividing* two positive numbers always results in a positive answer.
7. *Dividing* one positive number by one negative number always results
   in a negative answer.
8. *Dividing* two negative numbers always results in a positive answer.

SQUARES AND SQUARE ROOTS

Two common calculations you will have to carry out in the following statistical tests are squares and square roots. The *square* of a number is quite
simply that number multiplied by itself and is expressed by a small 2 thus:

8^2

This means that you multiply 8 by 8. So whenever you see the small 2
beside a number, you simply multiply that number by itself. The answer
you will obtain will always be a positive number, since if you square $+8$
you multiply $+8 \times +8$ which will give you $+64$, while if you square -8, you
multiply -8×-8 which will still give you $+64$, since multiplying two negative
numbers always gives a positive number.

The *square root* of a number is actually the opposite of the square, in
that the square root of any given number is a number which multiplied by
itself gives the number you already have. It is expressed by the symbol $\sqrt{}$.
Therefore $\sqrt{25} = 5$, since $5 \times 5 = 25$. While your calculator will almost
certainly have a square root function (which you should not hesitate to
use), this is a good example of an occasion when you should be 'eyeballing'
the result. For example, while you cannot easily work out in your head
what the square root of 14 is, you do know that it must be somewhere
between 3 and 4, since 3 is the square of 9 and 4 is the square root of 16; if
you come out with something larger or smaller, something has gone wrong
somewhere!

In many of the formulae in this book, you will find that the square root
sign extends over more than one number, e.g. $\sqrt{45 + 19} = \sqrt{64} = 8$. *Do*

make sure that you complete *all* the calculations under the square root symbol before computing the square root.

ROUNDING UP DECIMAL PLACES

When using decimals in fairly complicated calculations, you can often end up with a whole row of figures to the right of the decimal point. To continue your calculations with all these numbers is both cumbersome and unnecessarilly accurate. Therefore, it is easier to limit the number of figures to the right of the decimal point to 2 or 3. In order to do this correctly, we do not simply chop off the excess figures, but *round them up*.

This is done by starting with the figure on the extreme right of the decimal point. If this figure is equal to 5 or larger, then the number to its immediate left is increased by 1. If the end figure is less than 5, then the number to its left remains the same:

e.g. 9.14868125 becomes
     9.1486813

If you wish to drop the 3, the same rule applies, so that the above decimal becomes:

9.149681

If you wish to cut down the number of decimal places to 2, the process is:

9.148681 becomes
9.14868   which becomes
9.1487   which becomes
9.149   which becomes
9.15

While this process is relatively straightforward in the above example, look at the following decimal number, which we wish to round up to 2 places:

7.19498

Here, dropping the last number changes the 9 to a 10, and this automatically changes the 4 to 5 which in turn changes the next 9 into a 10, such that the end result is 7.2 — even though we were rounding up to 2 decimal places, thus:

7.19498 becomes
7.195   which becomes
7.2

Throughout this book, the figures have been rounded to 3 decimal places. If you have chosen to round up to 2 decimal places throughout the calculations, you will find that the end result is slightly different. Don't worry about this unless there is a massive discrepancy which will probably mean that something has gone wrong somewhere in your calculations.

Appendix 2

Statistical probability tables

Table A2.1 Critical values of χ^2 at various levels of probability (For your χ^2 value to be significant at a particular probability level, it should be *equal to* or *larger* than the critical values associated with the df in your study.)

df	Level of significance for a two-tailed test				
	.10	.05	.02	.01	.001
1	2.71	3.84	5.41	6.64	10.83
2	4.60	5.99	7.82	9.21	13.82
3	6.25	7.82	9.84	11.34	16.27
4	7.78	9.49	11.67	13.28	18.46
5	9.24	11.07	13.39	15.09	20.52
6	10.64	12.59	15.03	16.81	22.46
7	12.02	14.07	16.62	18.48	24.32
8	13.36	15.51	18.17	20.09	26.12
9	14.68	16.92	19.68	21.67	27.88
10	15.99	18.31	21.16	23.21	29.59
11	17.28	19.68	22.62	24.72	31.26
12	18.55	21.03	24.05	26.22	32.91
13	19.81	22.36	25.47	27.69	34.53
14	21.06	23.68	26.87	29.14	36.12
15	22.31	25.00	28.26	30.58	37.70
16	23.54	26.30	29.63	32.00	39.29
17	24.77	27.59	31.00	33.41	40.75
18	25.99	28.87	32.35	34.80	42.31
19	27.20	30.14	33.69	36.19	43.82
20	28.41	31.41	35.02	37.57	45.32
21	29.62	32.67	36.34	38.93	46.80
22	30.81	33.92	37.66	40.29	48.27
23	32.01	35.17	38.97	41.64	49.73
24	33.20	36.42	40.27	42.98	51.18
25	34.38	37.65	41.57	44.31	52.62
26	35.56	38.88	42.86	45.64	54.05
27	36.74	40.11	44.14	46.97	55.48
28	37.92	41.34	45.42	48.28	56.89
29	39.09	42.56	46.69	49.59	58.30
30	40.26	43.77	47.96	50.89	59.70

NB If you have a one-tailed hypothesis, look up your value as usual and simply *halve* the associated *P* value shown for a two-tailed hypothesis.

Table A2.2 Critical values of T (Wilcoxon test) at various levels of probability (For your T value to be significant at a particular probability level, it should be *equal to* or *less* than critical values associated with the N in your study)

Level of significance for one-tailed test					Level of significance for one-tailed test			
.05	.025	.01	.005		.05	.025	.01	.005
Level of significance for two-tailed test					Level of significance for two-tailed test			
N	.10	.05	.02	.01	N	.10	.05	.02	.01
5	1	—	—	—	28	130	117	102	92
6	2	1	—	—	29	141	127	111	100
7	4	2	0	—	30	152	137	120	109
8	6	4	2	0	31	163	148	130	118
9	8	6	3	2	32	175	159	141	128
10	11	8	5	3	33	188	171	151	138
11	14	11	7	5	34	201	183	162	149
12	17	14	10	7	35	214	195	174	160
13	21	17	13	10	36	228	208	186	171
14	26	21	16	13	37	242	222	198	183
15	30	25	20	16	38	256	235	211	195
16	36	30	24	19	39	271	250	224	208
17	41	35	28	23	40	287	264	238	221
18	47	40	33	28	41	303	279	252	234
19	54	46	38	32	42	319	295	267	248
20	60	52	43	37	43	336	311	281	262
21	68	59	49	43	44	353	327	297	277
22	75	66	56	49	45	371	344	313	292
23	83	73	62	55	46	389	361	329	307
24	92	81	69	61	47	408	379	345	323
25	101	90	77	68	48	427	397	362	339
26	110	98	85	76	49	446	415	380	356
27	120	107	93	84	50	466	434	398	373

Dashes in the table indicate that no decision is possible at the stated level of significance.

Table A2.3 Critical values of χ_r^2 (Friedman test) at various levels of probability. (For your χ_r^2 value to be significant at a particular probability level, it should be equal to or *larger* than the critical values associated with the *C* and *N* in your study)

a. Critical values for three conditions (C = 3)

χ_r^2	p	χ_r^2	p	χ_r^2	p	χ_r^2	p	χ_r^2	p	χ_r^2	p	χ_r^2	p	χ_r^2	p
	N = 2		N = 3		N = 4		N = 5		N = 6		N = 7		N = 8		N = 9
.000	1.000	.000	1.000	.0	1.000	.00	1.000	.000	1.000	.00	1.000	.00	1.000	.000	1.000
.833	.944	.667	.944	.4	.931	.33	.954	.286	.956	.25	.964	.25	.967	.222	.971
.500	.528	.2	.653	1.0	.740	.657	.768	.75	.794	.794	.814
2.000	.361	2.0	.431	1.6	.522	1.33	.570	.620	1.00	.654	.889	.865
4.667	.194	3.5	.273	2.8	.367	2.33	.430	2.000	.486	1.75	.531	1.556	.569
6.000	.028	4.5	.125	3.6	.182	3.00	.252	2.571	.305	2.25	.355	2.000	.398
		6.0	.069	4.8	.124	4.00	.184	3.429	.237	3.00	.285	2.667	.328
		6.5	.042	5.2	.093	4.33	.142	3.714	.192	3.25	.236	2.889	.278
		8.0	.0046	6.4	.039	5.33	.072	4.571	.112	4.00	.149	3.556	.187
				7.6	.024	6.33	.052	5.429	.085	4.75	.120	4.222	.154
				8.4	.0085	7.00	.029	6.000	.052	5.25	.079	4.667	.107
				10.0	.0077	8.33	.012	7.143	.027	6.25	.047	5.556	.069
						9.00	.0081	7.714	.021	6.75	.038	6.000	.057
						9.33	.0055	8.000	.016	7.00	.030	6.222	.048
						10.33	.0017	8.857	.0084	7.75	.018	6.889	.031
						12.00	.00013	10.286	.0036	9.00	.0099	8.000	.019
								10.571	.0027	9.25	.0080	8.222	.016
								11.143	.0012	9.75	.0048	8.667	.010
								12.286	.00032	10.75	.0024	9.556	.0060
								14.000	.000021	12.00	.0011	10.667	.0035
										12.25	.00086	10.889	.0029
										13.00	.00026	11.556	.0013
										14.25	.000061	12.667	.00066
										16.00	.0000036	13.556	.00035
												14.000	.00020
												14.222	.000097
												14.889	.000054
												16.222	.000011
												18.000	.0000006

Table A2.3 (contd) Critical values of χ_r^2 (Friedman test) (For your χ_r^2 value to be significant at a particular probability level, it should be *equal to* or *larger* than the critical values associated with the C and N in your study.)
b. Critical values for four conditions ($C = 4$)

$N = 2$		$N = 3$		$N = 4$			
χ_r^2	p	χ_r^2	p	χ_r^2	p	χ_r^2	p
.0	1.000	.0	1.000	.0	1.000	5.7	.141
.6	.958	.6	.958	.3	.992	6.0	.105
1.2	.834	1.0	.910	.6	.928	6.3	.094
1.8	.792	1.8	.727	.9	.900	6.6	.077
2.4	.625	2.2	.608	1.2	.800	6.9	.068
3.0	.542	2.6	.524	1.5	.754	7.2	.054
3.6	.458	3.4	.446	1.8	.677	7.5	.052
4.2	.375	3.8	.342	2.1	.649	7.8	.036
4.8	.208	4.2	.300	2.4	.524	8.1	.033
5.4	.167	5.0	.207	2.7	.508	8.4	.019
6.0	.042	5.4	.175	3.0	.432	8.7	.014
		5.8	.148	3.3	.389	9.3	.012
		6.6	.075	3.6	.355	9.6	.0069
		7.0	.054	3.9	.324	9.9	.0062
		7.4	.033	4.5	.242	10.2	.0027
		8.2	.017	4.8	.200	10.8	.0016
		9.0	.0017	5.1	.190	11.1	.00094
				5.4	.158	12.0	.000072

NB These values are all for a two-tailed test only.

Table A2.4 Critical values of L (Page's L trend test) at various levels of probability (For your L value to be significant at a particular probability level, it should be *equal to* or *larger* than the critical values associated with the C and N in your study)

N	C (no. of conditions)				$p <$
	3	4	5	6	
2	—	—	109	178	.001
	—	60	106	173	.01
	28	58	103	166	.05
3	—	89	160	260	.001
	42	87	155	252	.01
	41	84	150	244	.05
4	56	117	210	341	.001
	55	114	204	331	.01
	54	111	197	321	.05
5	70	145	259	420	.001
	68	141	251	409	.01
	66	137	244	397	.05
6	83	172	307	499	.001
	81	167	299	486	.01
	79	163	291	474	.05
7	96	198	355	577	.001
	93	193	346	563	.01
	91	189	338	550	.05
8	109	225	403	655	.001
	106	220	393	640	.01
	104	214	384	625	.05
9	121	252	451	733	.001
	119	246	441	717	.01
	116	240	431	701	.05
10	134	278	499	811	.001
	131	272	487	793	.01
	128	266	477	777	.05
11	147	305	546	888	.001
	144	298	534	869	.01
	141	292	523	852	.05
12	160	331	593	965	.001
	156	324	581	946	.01
	153	317	570	928	.05

NB These values are for a one-tailed test only.

Table A2.5 Critical values of t (related and unrelated t tests) at various levels of probability (for your t value to be significant at a particular probability level, it should be *equal to* or *larger* than the critical values associated with the df in your study)

	Level of significance for one-tailed test					
	.10	.05	.025	.01	.005	.0005
	Level of significance for two-tailed test					
df	.20	.10	.05	.02	.01	.001
1	3.078	6.314	12.706	31.821	63.657	636.619
2	1.886	2.920	4.303	6.965	9.925	31.598
3	1.638	2.353	3.182	4.541	5.841	12.941
4	1.533	2.132	2.776	3.747	4.604	8.610
5	1.476	2.015	2.571	3.365	4.032	6.859
6	1.440	1.943	2.447	3.143	3.707	5.959
7	1.415	1.895	2.365	2.998	3.499	5.405
8	1.397	1.860	2.306	2.896	3.355	5.041
9	1.383	1.833	2.262	2.821	3.250	4.781
10	1.372	1.812	2.228	2.764	3.169	4.587
11	1.363	1.796	2.201	2.718	3.106	4.437
12	1.356	1.782	2.179	2.681	3.055	4.318
13	1.350	1.771	2.160	2.650	3.012	4.221
14	1.345	1.761	2.145	2.624	2.977	4.140
15	1.341	1.753	2.131	2.602	2.947	4.073
16	1.337	1.746	2.120	2.583	2.921	4.015
17	1.333	1.740	2.110	2.567	2.898	3.965
18	1.330	1.734	2.101	2.552	2.878	3.922
19	1.328	1.729	2.093	2.539	2.861	3.883
20	1.325	1.725	2.086	2.528	2.845	3.850
21	1.323	1.721	2.080	2.518	2.831	3.819
22	1.321	1.717	2.074	2.508	2.819	3.792
23	1.319	1.714	2.069	2.500	2.807	3.767
24	1.318	1.711	2.064	2.492	2.797	3.745
25	1.316	1.708	2.060	2.485	2.787	3.725
26	1.315	1.706	2.056	2.479	2.779	3.707
27	1.314	1.703	2.052	2.473	2.771	3.690
28	1.313	1.701	2.048	2.467	2.763	3.674
29	1.311	1.699	2.045	2.462	2.756	3.659
30	1.310	1.697	2.042	2.457	2.750	3.646
40	1.303	1.684	2.021	2.423	2.704	3.551
60	1.296	1.671	2.000	2.390	2.660	3.460
120	1.289	1.658	1.980	2.358	2.617	3.373
∞	1.282	1.645	1.960	2.326	2.576	3.291

NB When there is no exact df use the next lowest number, except for very large dfs (well over 120), when you should use the infinity row. This is marked ∞.

Table A2.6 Critical values of F (anovas) at various levels of probability. (For your F value to be significant at a particular probability level, it should be *equal to* or *larger* than the critical values associated with v_1 and v_2 in your study)

a. Critical value of F at $< p$ .05

v_2	v_1											
	1	2	3	4	5	6	7	8	10	12	24	∞
1	161.4	199.5	215.7	224.6	230.2	234.0	236.8	238.9	241.9	243.9	249.0	254.3
2	18.5	19.0	19.2	19.2	19.3	19.3	19.4	19.4	19.4	19.4	19.5	19.5
3	10.13	9.55	9.28	9.12	9.01	8.94	8.89	8.85	8.79	8.74	8.64	8.53
4	7.71	6.94	6.59	6.39	6.26	6.16	6.09	6.04	5.96	5.91	5.77	5.63
5	6.61	5.79	5.41	5.19	5.05	4.95	4.88	4.82	4.74	4.68	4.53	4.36
6	5.99	5.14	4.76	4.53	4.39	4.28	4.21	4.15	4.06	4.00	3.84	3.67
7	5.59	4.74	4.35	4.12	3.97	3.87	3.79	3.73	3.64	3.57	3.41	3.23
8	5.32	4.46	4.07	3.84	3.69	3.58	3.50	3.44	3.35	3.28	3.12	2.93
9	5.12	4.26	3.86	3.63	3.48	3.37	3.29	3.23	3.14	3.07	2.90	2.71
10	4.96	4.10	3.71	3.48	3.33	3.22	3.14	3.07	2.98	2.91	2.74	2.54
11	4.84	3.98	3.59	3.36	3.20	3.09	3.01	2.95	2.85	2.79	2.61	2.40
12	4.75	3.89	3.49	3.26	3.11	3.00	2.91	2.85	2.75	2.69	2.51	2.30
13	4.67	3.81	3.41	3.18	3.03	2.92	2.83	2.77	2.67	2.60	2.42	2.21
14	4.60	3.74	3.34	3.11	2.96	2.85	2.76	2.70	2.60	2.53	2.35	2.13
15	4.54	3.68	3.29	3.06	2.90	2.79	2.71	2.64	2.54	2.48	2.29	2.07
16	4.49	3.63	3.24	3.01	2.85	2.74	2.66	2.59	2.49	2.42	2.24	2.01
17	4.45	3.59	3.20	2.96	2.81	2.70	2.61	2.55	2.45	2.38	2.19	1.96
18	4.41	3.55	3.16	2.93	2.77	2.66	2.58	2.51	2.41	2.34	2.15	1.92
19	4.38	3.52	3.13	2.90	2.74	2.63	2.54	2.48	2.38	2.31	2.11	1.88
20	4.35	3.49	3.10	2.87	2.71	2.60	2.51	2.45	2.35	2.28	2.08	1.84
21	4.32	3.47	3.07	2.84	2.68	2.57	2.49	2.42	2.32	2.25	2.05	1.81
22	4.30	3.44	3.05	2.82	2.66	2.55	2.46	2.40	2.30	2.23	2.03	1.78
23	4.28	3.42	3.03	2.80	2.64	2.53	2.44	2.37	2.27	2.20	2.00	1.76
24	4.26	3.40	3.01	2.78	2.62	2.51	2.42	2.36	2.25	2.18	1.98	1.73
25	4.24	3.39	2.99	2.76	2.60	2.49	2.40	2.34	2.24	2.16	1.96	1.71
26	4.23	3.37	2.98	2.74	2.59	2.47	2.39	2.32	2.22	2.15	1.95	1.69
27	4.21	3.35	2.96	2.73	2.57	2.46	2.37	2.31	2.20	2.13	1.93	1.67
28	4.20	3.34	2.95	2.71	2.56	2.45	2.36	2.29	2.19	2.12	1.91	1.65
29	4.18	3.33	2.93	2.70	2.55	2.43	2.35	2.28	2.18	2.10	1.90	1.64
30	4.17	3.32	2.92	2.69	2.53	2.42	2.33	2.27	2.16	2.09	1.89	1.62
32	4.15	3.29	2.90	2.67	2.51	2.40	2.31	2.24	2.14	2.07	1.86	1.59
34	4.13	3.28	2.88	2.65	2.49	2.38	2.29	2.23	2.12	2.05	1.84	1.57
36	4.11	3.26	2.87	2.63	2.48	2.36	2.28	2.21	2.11	2.03	1.82	1.55
38	4.10	3.24	2.85	2.62	2.46	2.35	2.26	2.19	2.09	2.02	1.81	1.53
40	4.08	3.23	2.84	2.61	2.45	2.34	2.25	2.18	2.08	2.00	1.79	1.51
60	4.00	3.15	2.76	2.53	2.37	2.25	2.17	2.10	1.99	1.92	1.70	1.39
120	3.92	3.07	2.68	2.45	2.29	2.18	2.09	2.02	1.91	1.83	1.61	1.25
∞	3.84	3.00	2.60	2.37	2.21	2.10	2.01	1.94	1.83	1.75	1.52	1.00

NB When there is no exact number for the df, use the next lowest number. For very large dfs (well over 120) you should use the row for infinity. This is indicated ∞.

These values are all for a two-tailed test only

Table A2.6 (contd) Critical values of F (anovas) at various levels of probability. (For your F value to be significant at a particular probability level, it should be *equal to* or *larger* than the critical values associated with v_1 and v_2 in your study)
b. Critical values of F at $p < .025$

						v_1						
v_2	1	2	3	4	5	6	7	8	10	12	24	∞
1	648	800	864	900	922	937	948	957	969	977	997	1018
2	38.5	39.0	39.2	39.2	39.3	39.3	39.4	39.4	39.4	39.4	39.5	39.5
3	17.4	16.0	15.4	15.1	14.9	14.7	14.6	14.5	14.4	14.3	14.1	13.9
4	12.22	10.65	9.98	9.60	9.36	9.20	9.07	8.98	8.84	8.75	8.51	8.26
5	10.01	8.43	7.76	7.39	7.15	6.98	6.85	6.76	6.62	6.52	6.28	6.02
6	8.81	7.26	6.60	6.23	5.99	5.82	5.70	5.60	5.46	5.37	5.12	4.85
7	8.07	6.54	5.89	5.52	5.29	5.12	4.99	4.90	4.76	4.67	4.42	4.14
8	7.57	6.06	5.42	5.05	4.82	4.65	4.53	4.43	4.30	4.20	3.95	3.67
9	7.21	5.71	5.08	4.72	4.48	4.32	4.20	4.10	3.96	3.87	3.61	3.33
10	6.94	5.46	4.83	4.47	4.24	4.07	3.95	3.85	3.72	3.62	3.37	3.08
11	6.72	5.26	4.63	4.28	4.04	3.88	3.76	3.66	3.53	3.43	3.17	2.88
12	6.55	5.10	4.47	4.12	3.89	3.73	3.61	3.51	3.37	3.28	3.02	2.72
13	6.41	4.97	4.35	4.00	3.77	3.60	3.48	3.39	3.25	3.15	2.89	2.60
14	6.30	4.86	4.24	3.89	3.66	3.50	3.38	3.29	3.15	3.05	2.79	2.49
15	6.20	4.76	4.15	3.80	3.58	3.41	3.29	3.20	3.06	2.96	2.70	2.40
16	6.12	4.69	4.08	3.73	3.50	3.34	3.22	3.12	2.99	2.89	2.63	2.32
17	6.04	4.62	4.01	3.66	3.44	3.28	3.16	3.06	2.92	2.82	2.56	2.25
18	5.98	4.56	3.95	3.61	3.38	3.22	3.10	3.01	2.87	2.77	2.50	2.19
19	5.92	4.51	3.90	3.56	3.33	3.17	3.05	2.96	2.82	2.72	2.45	2.13
20	5.87	4.46	3.86	3.51	3.29	3.13	3.01	2.91	2.77	2.68	2.41	2.09
21	5.83	4.42	3.82	3.48	3.25	3.09	2.97	2.87	2.73	2.64	2.37	2.04
22	5.79	4.38	3.78	3.44	3.22	3.05	2.93	2.84	2.70	2.60	2.33	2.00
23	5.75	4.35	3.75	3.41	3.18	3.02	2.90	2.81	2.67	2.57	2.30	1.97
24	5.72	4.32	3.72	3.38	3.15	2.99	2.87	2.78	2.64	2.54	2.27	1.94
25	5.69	4.29	3.69	3.35	3.13	2.97	2.85	2.75	2.61	2.51	2.24	1.91
26	5.66	4.27	3.67	3.33	3.10	2.94	2.82	2.73	2.59	2.49	2.22	1.88
27	5.63	4.24	3.65	3.31	3.08	2.92	2.80	2.71	2.57	2.47	2.19	1.85
28	5.61	4.22	3.63	3.29	3.06	2.90	2.78	2.69	2.55	2.45	2.17	1.83
29	5.59	4.20	3.61	3.27	3.04	2.88	2.76	2.67	2.53	2.43	2.15	1.81
30	5.57	4.18	3.59	3.25	3.03	2.87	2.75	2.65	2.51	2.41	2.14	1.79
32	5.53	4.15	3.56	3.22	3.00	2.84	2.72	2.62	2.48	2.38	2.10	1.75
34	5.50	4.12	3.53	3.19	2.97	2.81	2.69	2.59	2.45	2.35	2.08	1.72
36	5.47	4.09	3.51	3.17	2.94	2.79	2.66	2.57	2.43	2.33	2.05	1.69
38	5.45	4.07	3.48	3.15	2.92	2.76	2.64	2.55	2.41	2.31	2.03	1.66
40	5.42	4.05	3.46	3.13	2.90	2.74	2.62	2.53	2.39	2.29	2.01	1.64
60	5.29	3.93	3.34	3.01	2.79	2.63	2.51	2.41	2.27	2.17	1.88	1.48
120	5.15	3.80	3.23	2.89	2.67	2.52	2.39	2.30	2.16	2.05	1.76	1.31
∞	5.02	3.69	3.12	2.79	2.57	2.41	2.29	2.19	2.05	1.94	1.64	1.00

NB When there is no exact number for the df, use the next lowest number. For very large dfs (i.e. well over 120) you should use the row for infinity, marked ∞.

These values are all for a two-tailed test only.

Table A2.6 (contd) Critical values of F (anovas) at various levels of probability. (For your F value to be significant at a particular probability level, it should be *equal to* or *larger* than the critical values associated with v_1 and v_2 in your study)

c. Critical values of F at $p < .01$

v_2						v_1						
	1	2	3	4	5	6	7	8	10	12	24	∞
1	4052	5000	5403	5625	5764	5859	5928	5981	6056	6106	6235	6366
2	98.5	99.0	99.2	99.2	99.3	99.3	99.4	99.4	99.4	99.4	99.5	99.5
3	34.1	30.8	29.5	28.7	28.2	27.9	27.7	27.5	27.2	27.1	26.6	26.1
4	21.2	18.0	16.7	16.0	15.5	15.2	15.0	14.8	14.5	14.4	13.9	13.5
5	16.26	13.27	12.06	11.39	10.97	10.67	10.46	10.29	10.05	9.89	9.47	9.02
6	13.74	10.92	9.78	9.15	8.75	8.47	8.26	8.10	7.87	7.72	7.31	6.88
7	12.25	9.55	8.45	7.85	7.46	7.19	6.99	6.84	6.62	6.47	6.07	5.65
8	11.26	8.65	7.59	7.01	6.63	6.37	6.18	6.03	5.81	5.67	5.28	4.86
9	10.56	8.02	6.99	6.42	6.06	5.80	5.61	5.47	5.26	5.11	4.73	4.31
10	10.04	7.56	6.55	5.99	5.64	5.39	5.20	5.06	4.85	4.71	4.33	3.91
11	9.65	7.21	6.22	5.67	5.32	5.07	4.89	4.74	4.54	4.40	4.02	3.60
12	9.33	6.93	5.95	5.41	5.06	4.82	4.64	4.50	4.30	4.16	3.78	3.36
13	9.07	6.70	5.74	5.21	4.86	4.62	4.44	4.30	4.10	3.96	3.59	3.17
14	8.86	6.51	5.56	5.04	4.70	4.46	4.28	4.14	3.94	3.80	3.43	3.00
15	8.68	6.36	5.42	4.89	4.56	4.32	4.14	4.00	3.80	3.67	3.29	2.87
16	8.53	6.23	5.29	4.77	4.44	4.20	4.03	3.89	3.69	3.55	3.18	2.75
17	8.40	6.11	5.18	4.67	4.34	4.10	3.93	3.79	3.59	3.46	3.08	2.65
18	8.29	6.01	5.09	4.58	4.25	4.01	3.84	3.71	3.51	3.37	3.00	2.57
19	8.18	5.93	5.01	4.50	4.17	3.94	3.77	3.63	3.43	3.30	2.92	2.49
20	8.10	5.85	4.94	4.43	4.10	3.87	3.70	3.56	3.37	3.23	2.86	2.42
21	8.02	5.78	4.87	4.37	4.04	3.81	3.64	3.51	3.31	3.17	2.80	2.36
22	7.95	5.72	4.82	4.31	3.99	3.76	3.59	3.45	3.26	3.12	2.75	2.31
23	7.88	5.66	4.76	4.26	3.94	3.71	3.54	3.41	3.21	3.07	2.70	2.26
24	7.82	5.61	4.72	4.22	3.90	3.67	3.50	3.36	3.17	3.03	2.66	2.21
25	7.77	5.57	4.68	4.18	3.86	3.63	3.46	3.32	3.13	2.99	2.62	2.17
26	7.72	5.53	4.64	4.14	3.82	3.59	3.42	3.29	3.09	2.96	2.58	2.13
27	7.68	5.49	4.60	4.11	3.78	3.56	3.39	3.26	3.06	2.93	2.55	2.10
28	7.64	5.45	4.57	4.07	3.75	3.53	3.36	3.23	3.03	2.90	2.52	2.06
29	7.60	5.42	4.54	4.04	3.73	3.50	3.33	3.20	3.00	2.87	2.49	2.03
30	7.56	5.39	4.51	4.02	3.70	3.47	3.30	3.17	2.98	2.84	2.47	2.01
32	7.50	5.34	4.46	3.97	3.65	3.43	3.26	3.13	2.93	2.80	2.42	1.96
34	7.45	5.29	4.42	3.93	3.61	3.39	3.22	3.09	2.90	2.76	2.38	1.91
36	7.40	5.25	4.38	3.89	3.58	3.35	3.18	3.05	2.86	2.72	2.35	1.87
38	7.35	5.21	4.34	3.86	3.54	3.32	3.15	3.02	2.83	2.69	2.32	1.84
40	7.31	5.18	4.31	3.83	3.51	3.29	3.12	2.99	2.80	2.66	2.29	1.80
60	7.08	4.98	4.13	3.65	3.34	3.12	2.95	2.82	2.63	2.50	2.12	1.60
120	6.85	4.79	3.95	3.48	3.17	2.96	2.79	2.66	2.47	2.34	1.95	1.38
∞	6.63	4.61	3.78	3.32	3.02	2.80	2.64	2.51	2.32	2.18	1.79	1.00

NB When there is no exact number for the df, use the next lowest number. For very large dfs (i.e. well over 120) you should use the row for infinity, marked ∞.

These values are all for a two-tailed test only.

Table A2.6 (contd) Critical values of F (anovas) at various levels of probability. (For your F value to be significant at a particular probability level, it should be *equal to* or *larger* than the critical values associated with v_1 and v_2 in your study)

d. Critical values of F at $p < .001$

					v_1							
v_2	1	2	3	4	5	6	7	8	10	12	24	∞
1*4053	5000	5404	5625	5764	5859	5929	5981	6056	6107	6235	6366*
2 998.5	999.0	999.2	999.2	999.3	999.3	999.4	999.4	999.4	999.4	999.5	999.5
3 167.0	148.5	141.1	137.1	134.6	132.8	131.5	130.6	129.2	128.3	125.9	123.5
4 74.14	61.25	56.18	53.44	51.71	50.53	49.66	49.00	48.05	47.41	45.77	44.05
5 47.18	37.12	33.20	31.09	29.75	28.83	28.16	27.65	26.92	26.42	25.14	23.79
6 35.51	27.00	23.70	21.92	20.80	20.03	19.46	19.03	18.41	17.99	16.90	15.75
7 29.25	21.69	18.77	17.20	16.21	15.52	15.02	14.63	14.08	13.71	12.73	11.70
8 25.42	18.49	15.83	14.39	13.48	12.86	12.40	12.05	11.54	11.19	10.30	9.34
9 22.86	16.39	13.90	12.56	11.71	11.13	10.69	10.37	9.87	9.57	8.72	7.81
10 21.04	14.91	12.55	11.28	10.48	9.93	9.52	9.20	8.74	8.44	7.64	6.76
11 19.69	13.81	11.56	10.35	9.58	9.05	8.66	8.35	7.92	7.63	6.85	6.00
12 18.64	12.97	10.80	9.63	8.89	8.38	8.00	7.71	7.29	7.00	6.25	5.42
13 17.82	12.31	10.21	9.07	8.35	7.86	7.49	7.21	6.80	6.52	5.78	4.97
14 17.14	11.78	9.73	8.62	7.92	7.44	7.08	6.80	6.40	6.13	5.41	4.60
15 16.59	11.34	9.34	8.25	7.57	7.09	6.74	6.47	6.08	5.81	5.10	4.31
16 16.12	10.97	9.01	7.94	7.27	6.80	6.46	6.19	5.81	5.55	4.85	4.06
17 15.72	10.66	8.73	7.68	7.02	6.56	6.22	5.96	5.58	5.32	4.63	3.85
18 15.38	10.39	8.49	7.46	6.81	6.35	6.02	5.76	5.39	5.13	4.45	3.67
19 15.08	10.16	8.28	7.27	6.62	6.18	5.85	5.59	5.22	4.97	4.29	3.51
20 14.82	9.95	8.10	7.10	6.46	6.02	5.69	5.44	5.08	4.82	4.15	3.38
21 14.59	9.77	7.94	6.95	6.32	5.88	5.56	5.31	4.95	4.70	4.03	3.26
22 14.38	9.61	7.80	6.81	6.19	5.76	5.44	5.19	4.83	4.58	3.92	3.15
23 14.19	9.47	7.67	6.70	6.08	5.65	5.33	5.09	4.73	4.48	3.82	3.05
24 14.03	9.34	7.55	6.59	5.98	5.55	5.23	4.99	4.64	4.39	3.74	2.97
25 13.88	9.22	7.45	6.49	5.89	5.46	5.15	4.91	4.56	4.31	3.66	2.89
26 13.74	9.12	7.36	6.41	5.80	5.38	5.07	4.83	4.48	4.24	3.59	2.82
27 13.61	9.02	7.27	6.33	5.73	5.31	5.00	4.76	4.41	4.17	3.52	2.75
28 13.50	8.93	7.19	6.25	5.66	5.24	4.93	4.69	4.35	4.11	3.46	2.69
29 13.39	8.85	7.12	6.19	5.59	5.18	4.87	4.64	4.29	4.05	3.41	2.64
30 13.29	8.77	7.05	6.12	5.53	5.12	4.82	4.58	4.24	4.00	3.36	2.59
32 13.12	8.64	6.94	6.01	5.43	5.02	4.72	4.48	4.14	3.91	3.27	2.50
34 12.97	8.52	6.83	5.92	5.34	4.93	4.63	4.40	4.06	3.83	3.19	2.42
36 12.83	8.42	6.74	5.84	5.26	4.86	4.56	4.33	3.99	3.76	3.12	2.35
38 12.71	8.33	6.66	5.76	5.19	4.79	4.49	4.26	3.93	3.70	3.06	2.29
40 12.61	8.25	6.59	5.70	5.13	4.73	4.44	4.21	3.87	3.64	3.01	2.23
60 11.97	7.77	6.17	5.31	4.76	4.37	4.09	3.86	3.54	3.32	2.69	1.89
120 11.38	7.32	5.78	4.95	4.42	4.04	3.77	3.55	3.24	3.02	2.40	1.54
∞ 10.83	6.91	5.42	4.62	4.10	3.74	3.47	3.27	2.96	2.74	2.13	1.00

* Critical values to the right of $V_2 = 1$ should all be multiplied by 100, i.e. 4053 should be 40 5300.

NB When there is no exact number for the df, use the next lowest number. For very large dfs (i.e. well over 120) you should use the row for infinity, marked ∞.

These values are all for a two-tailed test only.

Table A2.7 Critical values of U (Mann-Whitney U test) at various levels of probability. (For your U value to be significant at a particular probability level, it should be *equal to* or *less* than the critical value associated with n_1 and n_2 in your study.)

a. Critical values of U for a one-tailed test at .005; two-tailed test at .01*

n_2										n_1										
	1	2	3	4	5	6	7	8	9	10	11	12	13	14	15	16	17	18	19	20
1	—	—	—	—	—	—	—	—	—	—	—	—	—	—	—	—	—	—	—	—
2	—	—	—	—	—	—	—	—	—	—	—	—	—	—	—	—	—	—	0	0
3	—	—	—	—	—	—	—	—	0	0	0	1	1	1	2	2	2	2	3	3
4	—	—	—	—	—	0	0	1	1	2	2	3	3	4	5	5	6	6	7	8
5	—	—	—	—	0	1	1	2	3	4	5	6	7	7	8	9	10	11	12	13
6	—	—	—	0	1	2	3	4	5	6	7	9	10	11	12	13	15	16	17	18
7	—	—	—	0	1	3	4	6	7	9	10	12	13	15	16	18	19	21	22	24
8	—	—	—	1	2	4	6	7	9	11	13	15	17	18	20	22	24	26	28	30
9	—	—	0	1	3	5	7	9	11	13	16	18	20	22	24	27	29	31	33	36
10	—	—	0	2	4	6	9	11	13	16	18	21	24	26	29	31	34	37	39	42
11	—	—	0	2	5	7	10	13	16	18	21	24	27	30	33	36	39	42	45	48
12	—	—	1	3	6	9	12	15	18	21	24	27	31	34	37	41	44	47	51	54
13	—	—	1	3	7	10	13	17	20	24	27	31	34	38	42	45	49	53	56	60
14	—	—	1	4	7	11	15	18	22	26	30	34	38	42	46	50	54	58	63	67
15	—	—	2	5	8	12	16	20	24	29	33	37	42	46	51	55	60	64	69	73
16	—	—	2	5	9	13	18	22	27	31	36	41	45	50	55	60	65	70	74	79
17	—	—	2	6	10	15	19	24	29	34	39	44	49	54	60	65	70	75	81	86
18	—	—	2	6	11	16	21	26	31	37	42	47	53	58	64	70	75	81	87	92
19	—	0	3	7	12	17	22	28	33	39	45	51	56	63	69	74	81	87	93	99
20	—	0	3	8	13	18	24	30	36	42	48	54	60	67	73	79	86	92	99	105

*Dashes in the table mean that no decision is possible for those n values at the given level of significance.

b. Critical values of U for a one-tailed test at .01; two-tailed test at .02*

n_2										n_1										
	1	2	3	4	5	6	7	8	9	10	11	12	13	14	15	16	17	18	19	20
1	—	—	—	—	—	—	—	—	—	—	—	—	—	—	—	—	—	—	—	—
2	—	—	—	—	—	—	—	—	—	—	—	—	0	0	0	0	0	0	1	1
3	—	—	—	—	—	—	—	0	0	1	1	1	2	2	2	3	3	4	4	5
4	—	—	—	—	0	1	1	2	3	3	4	5	5	6	7	7	8	9	9	10
5	—	—	—	0	1	2	3	4	5	6	7	8	9	10	11	12	13	14	15	16
6	—	—	—	1	2	3	4	6	7	8	9	11	12	13	15	16	18	19	20	22
7	—	—	0	1	3	4	6	7	9	11	12	14	16	17	19	21	23	24	26	28
8	—	—	0	2	4	6	7	9	11	13	15	17	20	22	24	26	28	30	32	34
9	—	—	1	3	5	7	9	11	14	16	18	21	23	26	28	31	33	36	38	40
10	—	—	1	3	6	8	11	13	16	19	22	24	27	30	33	36	38	41	44	47
11	—	—	1	4	7	9	12	15	18	22	25	28	31	34	37	41	44	47	50	53
12	—	—	2	5	8	11	14	17	21	24	28	31	35	38	42	46	49	53	56	60
13	—	0	2	5	9	12	16	20	23	27	31	35	39	43	47	51	55	59	63	67
14	—	0	2	6	10	13	17	22	26	30	34	38	43	47	51	56	60	65	69	73
15	—	0	3	7	11	15	19	24	28	33	37	42	47	51	56	61	66	70	75	80
16	—	0	3	7	12	16	21	26	31	36	41	46	51	56	61	66	71	76	82	87
17	—	0	4	8	13	18	23	28	33	38	44	49	55	60	66	71	77	82	88	93
18	—	0	4	9	14	19	24	30	36	41	47	53	59	65	70	76	82	88	94	100
19	—	1	4	9	15	20	26	32	38	44	50	56	63	69	75	82	88	94	101	107
20	—	1	5	10	16	22	28	34	40	47	53	60	67	73	80	87	93	100	107	114

*Dashes in the table mean that no decision is possible for those n values at the given level of significance.

Table A2.7 (contd) Critical values of U (Mann-Whitney U test) at various levels of probability. (For your U value to be significant at a particular probability level, it should be *equal to* or *less* than the critical value associated with n_1 and n_2 in your study.)

c. Critical values of U for a one-tailed test at .025; two-tailed test at .05*

								n_1												
n_2	1	2	3	4	5	6	7	8	9	10	11	12	13	14	15	16	17	18	19	20
1	—	—	—	—	—	—	—	—	—	—	—	—	—	—	—	—	—	—	—	—
2	—	—	—	—	—	—	—	—	0	0	0	0	1	1	1	1	1	2	2	2	2
3	—	—	—	—	0	1	1	2	2	3	3	4	4	5	5	6	6	7	7	8
4	—	—	—	0	1	2	3	4	4	5	6	7	8	9	10	11	11	12	13	13
5	—	—	0	1	2	3	5	6	7	8	9	11	12	13	14	15	17	18	19	20
6	—	—	1	2	3	5	6	8	10	11	13	14	16	17	19	21	22	24	25	27
7	—	—	1	3	5	6	8	10	12	14	16	18	20	22	24	26	28	30	32	34
8	—	0	2	4	6	8	10	13	15	17	19	22	24	26	29	31	34	36	38	41
9	—	0	2	4	7	10	12	15	17	20	23	26	28	31	34	37	39	42	45	48
10	—	0	3	5	8	11	14	17	20	23	26	29	33	36	39	42	45	48	52	55
11	—	0	3	6	9	13	16	19	23	26	30	33	37	40	44	47	51	55	58	62
12	—	1	4	7	11	14	18	22	26	29	33	37	41	45	49	53	57	61	65	69
13	—	1	4	8	12	16	20	24	28	33	37	41	45	50	54	59	63	67	72	76
14	—	1	5	9	13	17	22	26	31	36	40	45	50	55	59	64	67	74	78	83
15	—	1	5	10	14	19	24	29	34	39	44	49	54	59	64	70	75	80	85	90
16	—	1	6	11	15	21	26	31	37	42	47	53	59	64	70	75	81	86	92	98
17	—	2	6	11	17	22	28	34	39	45	51	57	63	67	75	81	87	93	99	105
18	—	2	7	12	18	24	30	36	42	48	55	61	67	74	80	86	93	99	106	112
19	—	2	7	13	19	25	32	38	45	52	58	65	72	78	85	92	99	106	113	119
20	—	2	8	13	20	27	34	41	48	55	62	69	76	83	90	98	105	112	119	127

*Dashes in the table mean that no decision is possible for those n values at the given level of significance.

d. Critical values of U for a one-tailed test at .05; two-tailed test at .10*

								n_1												
n_2	1	2	3	4	5	6	7	8	9	10	11	12	13	14	15	16	17	18	19	20
1	—	—	—	—	—	0	0	0	—	—	—	—	—	—	—	—	—	—	0	0
2	—	—	—	—	0	0	1	1	1	1	2	2	2	3	3	3	4	4	4
3	—	—	0	0	1	2	2	3	3	4	5	5	6	7	7	8	9	9	10	11
4	—	—	0	1	2	3	4	5	6	7	8	9	10	11	12	14	15	16	17	18
5	—	0	1	2	4	5	6	8	9	11	12	13	15	16	18	19	20	22	23	25
6	—	0	2	3	5	7	8	10	12	14	16	17	19	21	23	25	26	28	30	32
7	—	0	2	4	6	8	11	13	15	17	19	21	24	26	28	30	33	35	37	39
8	—	1	3	5	8	10	13	15	18	20	23	26	28	31	33	36	39	41	44	47
9	—	1	3	6	9	12	15	18	21	24	27	30	33	36	39	42	45	48	51	54
10	—	1	4	7	11	14	17	20	24	27	31	34	37	41	44	48	51	55	58	62
11	—	1	5	8	12	16	19	23	27	31	34	38	42	46	50	54	57	61	65	69
12	—	2	5	9	13	17	21	26	30	34	38	42	47	51	55	60	64	68	72	77
13	—	2	6	10	15	19	24	28	33	37	42	47	51	56	61	65	70	75	80	84
14	—	2	7	11	16	21	26	31	36	41	46	51	56	61	66	71	77	82	87	92
15	—	3	7	12	18	23	28	33	39	44	50	55	61	66	72	77	83	88	94	100
16	—	3	8	14	19	25	30	36	42	48	54	60	65	71	77	83	89	95	101	107
17	—	3	9	15	20	26	33	39	45	51	57	64	70	77	83	89	96	102	109	115
18	—	4	9	16	22	28	35	41	48	55	61	68	75	82	88	95	102	109	116	123
19	0	4	10	17	23	30	37	44	51	58	65	72	80	87	94	101	109	116	123	130
20	0	4	11	18	25	32	39	47	54	62	69	77	84	92	100	107	115	123	130	138

*Dashes in the table mean that no decision is possible for those n values at the given level of significance.

Table A2.8 Critical values of H (Kruskal-Wallis test) at various levels of probability. (For your H value to be significant at a particular probability level, it should be *equal to* or *larger* than the critical values associated with the ns in your study.)

Size of groups					Size of groups				
n_1	n_2	n_3	H	p	n_1	n_2	n_3	H	p
2	1	1	2.7000	.500	4	3	1	5.8333	.021
								5.2083	.050
2	2	1	3.6000	.200				5.0000	.057
								4.0556	.093
2	2	2	4.5714	.067				3.8889	.129
			3.7143	.200					
					4	3	2	6.4444	.008
3	1	1	3.2000	.300				6.3000	.011
								5.4444	.046
3	2	1	4.2857	.100				5.4000	.051
			3.8571	.133				4.5111	.098
								4.4444	.102
3	2	2	5.3572	.029					
			4.7143	.048	4	3	3	6.7455	.010
			4.5000	.067				6.7091	.013
			4.4643	.105				5.7909	.046
								5.7273	.050
3	3	1	5.1429	.043				4.7091	.092
			4.5714	.100				4.7000	.101
			4.0000	.129					
					4	4	1	6.6667	.010
3	3	2	6.2500	.011				6.1667	.022
			5.3611	.032				4.9667	.048
			5.1389	.061				4.8667	.054
			4.5556	.100				4.1667	.082
			4.2500	.121				4.0667	.102
3	3	3	7.2000	.004	4	4	2	7.0364	.006
			6.4889	.011				6.8727	.011
			5.6889	.029				5.4545	.046
			5.6000	.050				5.2364	.052
			5.0667	.086				4.5545	.098
			4.6222	.100				4.4455	.103
4	1	1	3.5714	.200	4	4	3	7.1439	.010
								7.1364	.011
4	2	1	4.8214	.057				5.5985	.049
			4.5000	.076				5.5758	.051
			4.0179	.114				4.5455	.099
								4.4773	.102
4	2	2	6.0000	.014					
			5.3333	.033	4	4	4	7.6538	.008
			5.1250	.052				7.5385	.011
			4.4583	.100				5.6923	.049
			4.1667	.105				5.6538	.054
								4.6539	.097
								4.5001	.104

NB These values are all for a two-tailed test only.

Table A2.8 (contd) Critical values of H (Kruskal-Wallis test) at various levels of probability. (For your H value to be significant at a particular probability level, it should be *equal to* or *larger* than the critical values associated with the ns in your study.)

Size of groups						Size of groups				
n_1	n_2	n_3	H	p		n_1	n_2	n_3	H	p
5	1	1	3.8571	.143		5	4	3	7.4449	.010
									7.3949	.011
5	2	1	5.2500	.036					5.6564	.049
			5.0000	.048					5.6308	.050
			4.4500	.071					4.5487	.099
			4.2000	.095					4.5231	.103
			4.0500	.119						
						5	4	4	7.7604	.009
5	2	2	6.5333	.008					7.7440	.011
			6.1333	.013					5.6571	.049
			5.1600	.034					5.6176	.050
			5.0400	.056					4.6187	.100
			4.3733	.090					4.5527	.102
			4.2933	.122						
						5	5	1	7.3091	.009
5	3	1	6.4000	.012					6.8364	.011
			4.9600	.048					5.1273	.046
			4.8711	.052					4.9091	.053
			4.0178	.095					4.1091	.086
			3.8400	.123					4.0364	.105
5	3	2	6.9091	.009		5	5	2	7.3385	.010
			6.8218	.010					7.2692	.010
			5.2509	.049					5.3385	.047
			5.1055	.052					5.2462	.051
			4.6509	.091					4.6231	.097
			4.4945	.101					4.5077	.100
5	3	3	7.0788	.009		5	5	3	7.5780	.010
			6.9818	.011					7.5429	.010
			5.6485	.049					5.7055	.046
			5.5152	.051					5.6264	.051
			4.5333	.097					4.5451	.100
			4.4121	.109					4.5363	.102
5	4	1	6.9545	.008		5	5	4	7.8229	.010
			6.8400	.011					7.7914	.010
			4.9855	.044					5.6657	.049
			4.8600	.056					5.6429	.050
			3.9873	.098					4.5229	.099
			3.9600	.102					4.5200	.101
5	4	2	7.2045	.009		5	5	5	8.0000	.009
			7.1182	.010					7.9800	.010
			5.2727	.049					7.7800	.049
			5.2682	.050					5.6600	.051
			4.5409	.098					4.5600	.100
			4.5182	.101					4.5000	.102

NB These values are all for a two-tailed test only.

Table A2.9 Critical values of S (Jonckheere trend test) at various levels of probability. (For your S value to be significant at a particular probability level, it should be *equal to* or *larger* than the critical values associated with C and n in your study.)

a. Significance level $p < .05$

	n								
C	2	3	4	5	6	7	8	9	10
3	10	17	24	33	42	53	64	76	88
4	14	26	38	51	66	82	100	118	138
5	20	34	51	71	92	115	140	166	194
6	26	44	67	93	121	151	184	219	256

b. Significance level $p < .01$

3	—	23	32	45	59	74	90	106	124
4	20	34	50	71	92	115	140	167	195
5	26	48	72	99	129	162	197	234	274
6	34	62	94	130	170	213	260	309	361

NB These values are all for a one-tailed test only.

Table A2.10 Critical values of r_s (Spearman test) at various levels of probability. (For your r_s value to be significant at a particular probability level, it should be *equal to* or *larger* than the critical values associated with N in your study.)

N (*number of subjects*)	Level of significance for one-tailed test			
	.05	.025	.01	.005
	Level of significance for two-tailed test			
	.10	.05	.02	.01
5	.900	1.000	1.000	—
6	.829	.886	.943	1.000
7	.714	.786	.893	.929
8	.643	.738	.833	.881
9	.600	.683	.783	.833
10	.564	.648	.746	.794
12	.506	.591	.712	.777
14	.456	.544	.645	.715
16	.425	.506	.601	.665
18	.399	.475	.564	.625
20	.377	.450	.534	.591
22	.359	.428	.508	.562
24	.343	.409	.485	.537
26	.329	.392	.465	.515
28	.317	.377	.448	.496
30	.306	.364	.432	.478

NB When there is no exact number of subjects use the next lowest number.

Table A2.11 Critical values of r (Pearson test) at various levels of probability. (For your r value to be significant at a particular probability level, it should be *equal to* or *larger* than the critical values associated with the df in your study.)

df = N − 2	Level of significance for one-tailed test				
	.05	.025	.01	.005	.0005
	Level of significance for two-tailed test				
	.10	.05	.02	.01	.001
1	.9877	.9969	.9995	.9999	1.0000
2	.9000	.9500	.9800	.9900	.9990
3	.8054	.8783	.9343	.9587	.9912
4	.7293	.8114	.8822	.9172	.9741
5	.6694	.7545	.8329	.8745	.9507
6	.6215	.7067	.7887	.8343	.9249
7	.5822	.6664	.7498	.7977	.8982
8	.5494	.6319	.7155	.7646	.8721
9	.5214	.6021	.6851	.7348	.8471
10	.4973	.5760	.6581	.7079	.8233
11	.4762	.5529	.6339	.6835	.8010
12	.4575	.5324	.6120	.6614	.7800
13	.4409	.5139	.5923	.6411	.7603
14	.4259	.4973	.5742	.6226	.7420
15	.4124	.4821	.5577	.6055	.7246
16	.4000	.4683	.5425	.5897	.7084
17	.3887	.4555	.5285	.5751	.6932
18	.3783	.4438	.5155	.5614	.6787
19	.3687	.4329	.5034	.5487	.6652
20	.3598	.4227	.4921	.5368	.6524
25	.3233	.3809	.4451	.4869	.5974
30	.2960	.3494	.4093	.4487	.5541
35	.2746	.3246	.3810	.4182	.5189
40	.2573	.3044	.3578	.3932	.4896
45	.2428	.2875	.3384	.3721	.4648
50	.2306	.2732	.3218	.3541	.4433
60	.2108	.2500	.2948	.3248	.4078
70	.1954	.2319	.2737	.3017	.3799
80	.1829	.2172	.2565	.2830	.3568
90	.1726	.2050	.2422	.2673	.3375
100	.1638	.1946	.2301	.2540	.3211

NB When there is no exact df use the next lowest number.

Table A2.12 Critical values of s (Kendall's coefficient of concordance) at various levels of probability. (For your s value to be significant at a particular probability level, it should be *equal to* or *larger* than the critical values associated with C and N in your study.)
a. Critical values of s at $p = 0.05$

C	$N = 3$	$N = 4$	$N = 5$	$N = 6$	$N = 7$
3	—	—	64.4	103.9	157.3
4	—	49.5	88.4	143.3	217.0
5	—	62.6	112.3	182.4	276.2
6	—	75.7	136.1	221.4	335.2
8	48.1	101.7	183.7	299.0	453.1
10	60.0	127.8	231.2	376.7	571.0
15	89.8	192.9	349.8	570.5	864.9
20	119.7	258.0	468.5	764.4	1158.7

b. Critical values of s at $p = 0.01$

C	$N = 3$	$N = 4$	$N = 5$	$N = 6$	$N = 7$
3	—	—	75.6	122.8	185.6
4	—	61.4	109.3	176.2	265.0
5	—	80.5	142.8	229.4	343.8
6	—	99.5	176.1	282.4	422.6
8	66.8	137.4	242.7	388.3	579.9
10	85.1	175.3	309.1	494.0	737.0
15	131.0	269.8	475.2	758.2	1129.5
20	177.0	364.2	641.2	1022.2	1521.9

NB The values are all for a one-tailed test only.
   A dash in the table means that no decision can be made at this level.

Appendix 3

Answers to activities in the text

Activity 1

1. 46	11. − 6
2. − 2	12. − 8
3. 43	13. − 48
4. 253	14. − 44
5. 65	15. 42
6. 49	16. − 48
7. 54	17. 45
8. 11	18. − 13
9. 104	19. + 7
10. 47	20. − 240

Activity 2

1. (a) Histogram

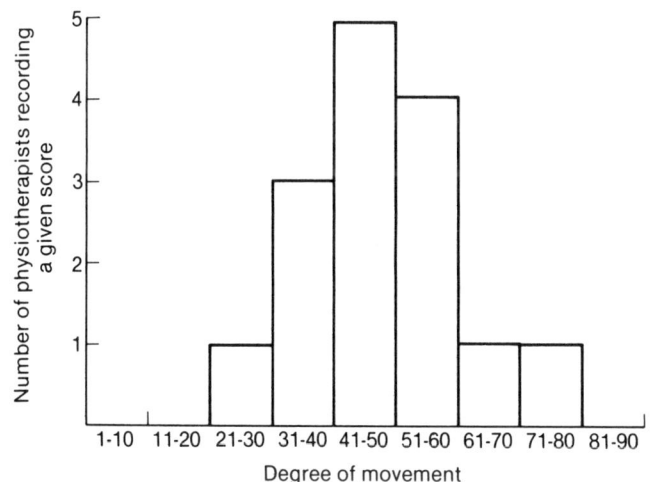

Fig. 34

(b) Bar graph

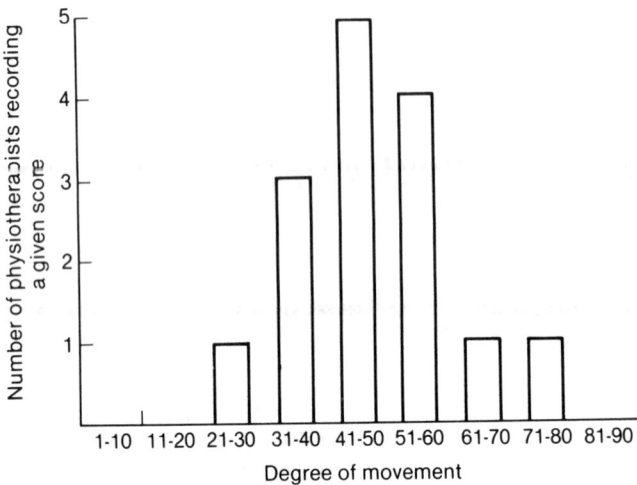

Fig. 35

(c) Frequency polygon

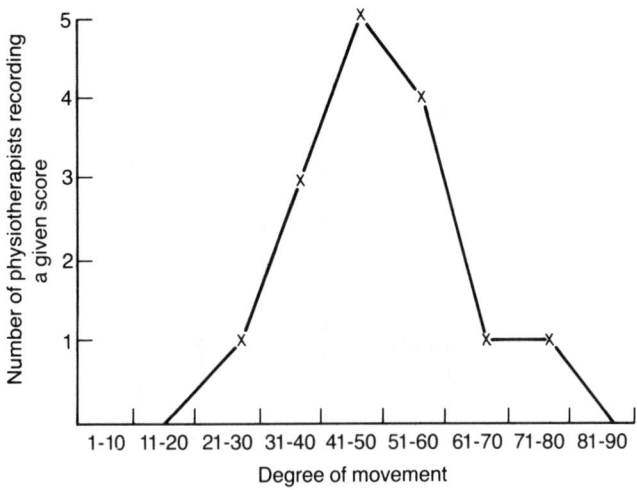

Fig. 36

2. Frequency polygon with reduced number of units along horizontal axis

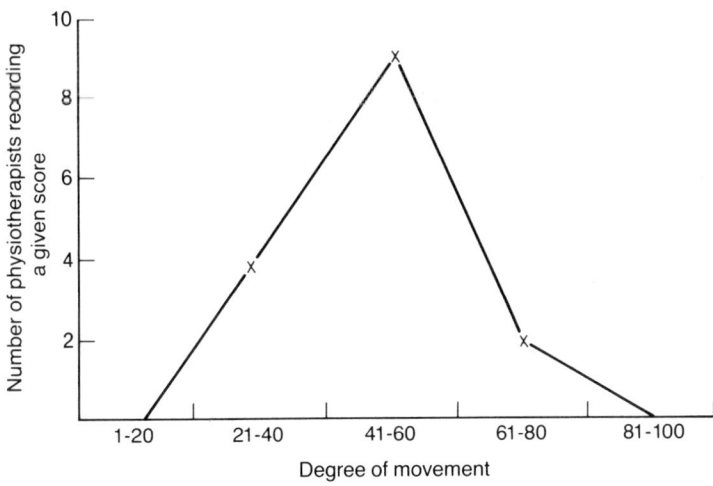

Fig. 37

Activity 3

1. (i) Mean   : 70.333
       Median : 76
       Mode   : 76
   (ii) Mean   : 28.667
       Median : 27
       Mode   : 17
   (iii) Mean : 50.1
       Median : 47.5
       Mode   : 43
2. Set of data (i) has the largest range of scores while (ii) has the smallest.

Activity 4

1. (i) Range   : 24
       Deviation : $14 - 19.444 = -5.444$
                   $9 - 19.444 = -10.444$
                   $21 - 19.444 = +1.556$
                   $23 - 19.444 = +3.556$
                   $18 - 19.444 = -1.444$
                   $17 - 19.444 = -2.444$
                   $33 - 19.444 = +13.556$
                   $28 - 19.444 = +8.556$
                   $12 - 19.444 = -7.444$

Variance : 474.221
Standard deviation : 7.259
(ii) Range : 33
Deviation : $71 - 67.571 = +3.429$
$50 - 67.571 = -17.571$
$48 - 67.571 = -19.571$
$64 - 67.571 = -3.571$
$80 - 67.571 = +12.429$
$81 - 67.571 = +13.429$
$79 - 67.571 = +11.429$
Variance : 1181.714
Standard deviation : 12.993

2. You might assess the reliability of the goniometer by taking several readings (e.g. 10) of the same joint on, say five different occasions. For each set of 10 readings you might calculate the mean and the median to assess the homogeneity or similarity of the scores. You might also wish to calculate the range and the standard deviation to find out how disparate the readings are.

Activity 5

1. (i) 95% of patients will have heart rates of between 66 and 98 during weeks 10–20 of pregnancy.
   (ii) 2.36% of patients will have heart rates of between 99 and 106.
   (iii) This patient comes in 0.135% of the population in terms of heart rate.

Activity 6

The two variables in each hypothesis are:
1. Age of patient (child or adolescent) and progress rate on traction.
2. Sex (male or female) and responsiveness to heat treatment.
3. Sex (male or female) and incidence of chest infections.
4. Type of clinic (outpatients or sports injuries) and recovery rate for leg fractures.
5. Type of training establishment (hospital-based or polytechnic-based) and professional competence.

Activity 7

The null hypotheses for these experimental hypotheses are:
1. There is no relationship between age of patient and progress rates on traction following leg fractures.
2. There is no relationship between the sex of arthritis patients and reponsiveness to heat treatment.

3. There is no relationship between sex of patient and incidence of chest infections following cardiothoracic surgery.
4. There is no relationship between type of physiotherapy clinic and recovery rates for leg fractures.
5. There is no relationship between type of training establishment and professional competence in physiotherapists.

Activity 8

1. IV = sex of patient.
   DV = tendency to complain about pain.
   IV manipulated by selecting one group of male patients and one group of female patients.
2. IV = type of walking aid.
   DV = mobility.
   IV manipulated by selecting a number of patients and deciding which walking aid each should receive.
3. IV = type of hospital.
   DV = absenteeism.
   IV manipulated by selecting one group of physiotherapists working in a psychiatric hospital and another group working in a general hospital.
4. IV = sex of patient.
   DV = degree of rapport.
   IV manipulated by selecting one group of male patients and one group of female patients.
5. IV = physiotherapy schools' entry requirements.
   DV = pass rate on CSP exam.
   IV manipulated by selecting a number of schools requiring 'A'-level physics and a number of schools not requiring 'A'-level physics.

Activity 9

Other possible explanations for a more tolerant attitude amongst these physiotherapists might be:
1. Simply the fact that they were a bit older and therefore a bit wiser, and perhaps as a result a bit more tolerant.
2. Experiencing a period of illness themselves which made them more aware of the patient's perspective.
3. Reading a book on attitude change.
4. Attending another sort of course.
Plus, of course, many other possible reasons.

Activity 10

Designs for hypotheses on page 45.

1. *Experimental Group* | *Pre-test measure of DV* | *Condition* | *Post-test measure of DV*
| Relaxation | Uniform | Relaxation

Control Group

| Relaxation | No Uniform | Relaxation

2. *Experimental Group* | *Pre-test measure of DV* | *Condition* | *Post-test measure of DV*

| Sympathy | Experience as hospital patient | Sympathy

Control Group

| Sympathy | No experience as hospital patient | Sympathy

3. *Experimental Group 1* | *Pre-test measure of DV* | *Condition* | *Post-test measure of DV*

| Motivation | < 5 years | Motivation

Experimental Group 2

| Motivation | > 10 years | Motivation

Activity 11

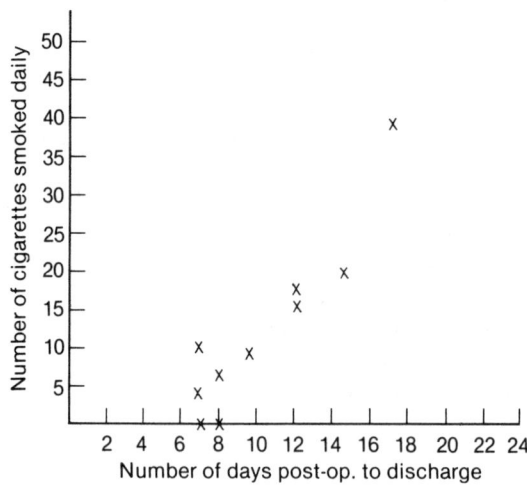

Fig. 38

Activity 12

1. (i) A positive correlation is predicted, with high scores on age being associated with high scores on recovery time. This would be represented by a general upward slope on a scattergram and a correlation coefficient of around $+1.0$.
    (ii) A negative correlation is predicted with high scores on distance being associated with low scores on attendance. This would be represented by a general downward slope on a scattergram and a correlation coefficient of around -1.0.
    (iii) A positive correlation is predicted with low scores on 'A'-levels being associated with low mock final exam scores. An upward slope and a correlation coefficient of around $+1.0$ would be anticipated.
    (iv) A negative correlation is predicted with high scores on fibre intake being associated with low scores on incidence of diverticulitis. A general downward slope and a correlation coefficient of around -1.0 would be predicted.
2. From strongest to weakest, the coefficients are:
    $-0.73 \qquad +0.61 \qquad -0.42 \qquad +0.21 \qquad -0.17 \qquad +0.09$

Activity 13

Some of the constant and random errors involved in these experiments are outlined below. You may have thought of many more.

H_1 Men are more likely to suffer respiratory complications following cardiothoracic surgery.

Constant error	Solution	Random error	Solution
1. Age of patient	Ensure both groups are of comparable age	1. Personality	Random selection of patients in each group
2. Nature of illness	Ensure both groups are being treated for the same complaint	2. Attitude	
3. Previous health	Establish comparability of previous health in both groups	3. Supportive family	
4. Previous relevant illnesses	Ensure both groups have had similar number/types of relevant illness	4. Biochemical make-up	
5. Smoker/Non-smoker	Ensure that no S in either group smokes	5. Inherent and undetected lung defects	
6. Vital capacity	Ensure that both groups have comparable vital capacity		

H_1 Outpatients' clinics achieve better recovery rates for leg fractures than specific sports injuries clinics.

Constant error	Solution	Random error	Solution
1. Age of patient	Ensure both groups of patients are of comparable age	1. Motivation of patient and therapist	
2. Nature of fracture	Ensure the type of fracture is the same in each case	2. Personality of patient and therapist	Randomly select
3. Fitness of patient	Ensure comparability of previous fitness in both groups	3. Attitude of patient and therapist	patients from each situation
4. Sex of patient	Ensure both groups comprise either all males, all females, or an equal number of each sex	4. Biochemical make-up	to take part in the experiment
5. Amount of time spent in treatment	Ensure that the amount of treatment is standardised in each case	5. Inherent and undetected bone defects	
6. Quality of treatment	Ensure that the type and quality of treatment is standardised in each case		

Activity 14

From greatest support to least:
$p = 0.01\%$ $p = 3\%$ $p = 5\%$ $p = 7\%$ $p = 15\%$ $p = 19\%$
Converted to a decimal:
$p = 0.0001$ $p = 0.03$ $p = 0.05$ $p = 0.07$ $p = 1.5$ $p = 1.9$

Activity 15

	% support for hypothesis	% probability that the results are due to chance
$p = 1\%$	99%	1%
$p = 7\%$	93%	7%
$p = 3\%$	97%	3%
$p = 5\%$	95%	5%
$p = 0.5\%$	99.5%	0.5%

Activity 16

The following are examples of nominal levels of measurement. Any variation on these which still involved allocating patients to a category is acceptable.

1. You might measure improvement in incontinence by asking the patient 'Did you experience any improvement following therapy?'
   Yes/No
2. This might be measured by categorising the patients as (a) either having had a chest infection or (b) *not* having had a chest infection.
3. You can assess whether or not a patient experienced an increased range of movement following manipulation by allocating him/her to either an 'Increase in movement' category or 'No increase in movement' category.
4. Patients could be classified as those who kept appointments and those who did not.
5. This might be assessed by asking patients to answer the following question: Did you find the treatment in the physiotherapy department to be:

good   [ ]   average   [ ]   poor   [ ]

Activity 17

Again, any variation on the answers suggested below is acceptable, as long as you are rank ordering your data according to the dimension you're interested in.

1. Improvement in incontinence might be measured by asking the patients to answer the following question:
   To what extent did your incontinence improve following therapy?

1	2	3	4	5
very much better	better	about the same	worse	very much worse

   Alternatively, you could rank order your subjects according to how much they improved.

2. This might be measured by assessing the patients along a scale of incidence of chest infection thus:
   The incidence of chest infection following breathing exercises was

1	2	3	4	5	6	7
very much reduced	much reduced	marginally reduced	the same	marginally increased	much increased	very much increased

   Similarly you could rank order the patients according to their incidence of chest infections.

3. Range of movement could be assessed by either rank ordering the subjects from the greatest increase in movement to the smallest increase, or alternatively you could use a point scale thus:

The increase in range of movement in the leg following manipulation was

1	2	3	4	5
very much greater	much greater	marginally greater	the same	worse

4. Likelihood of keeping appointments could be assessed by a point scale thus:

How likely is this patient to keep an appointment at the outpatients' clinic?

1	2	3	4	5
very likely	quite likely	not sure	quite unlikely	very unlikely

5. Assessing the quality of physiotherapy could be conducted along similar lines:

How would you rate the quality of the physiotherapy treatment you received?

1	2	3	4	5	6	7
excellent	very good	good	average	poor	very poor	appalling

Activity 18

1. You could measure incontinence on an interval/ratio scale simply by monitoring the number of times a patient was incontinent or the number of ccs of urine voided, accidentally.
2. Incidence of chest infection could be assessed by noting the number of times each patient suffered a chest problem following breathing exercises.
3. Range of movement could be measured in degrees.
4. The number of appointments kept and missed could be monitored for each patient.
5. You could ask the patients to rate the quality of physiotherapy by giving it marks out of 20 or 100.
6. (i) Accuracy of shooting an arrow at a target could be measured
   — on a nominal scale by counting up the number of hits and the number of misses.
   — on an ordinal scale by rank ordering each arrow's proximity to the target, giving a rank of 1 to the nearest etc.
   — on an interval/ratio scale by measuring the distance of each arrow from the target, in centimetres or inches.
   (ii) Improvement in mobility after a hip replacement operation could be measured:
   — on a nominal scale by classifying the patients according to whether they:

a. experienced an improvement in mobility or
b. experienced no improvement in mobility
— on a ordinal scale using a point scale thus:
What degree of improvement in mobility did this patient experience?

1	2	3	4	5
great improvement	some improvement	minimal improvement	no improvement	deteriorated

— on an interval/ratio scale by measuring the distance walked.
(iii) Relief of neck and arm pain following the use of a surgical collar could be measured:
— on a nominal scale by classifying patients according to whether they experienced pain relief, or did not experience pain relief.
— on an ordinal scale by using a point scale thus:
How much pain relief did you experience after wearing a surgical collar?

1	2	3	4	5
very great relief	great relief	some relief	no relief	deterioration

— on an interval/ratio scale by asking the patient the percentage of pain relief felt, e.g. was the pain about 50%/30%/25% less than it was prior to using the surgical collar?
7. (i) Nominal
(ii) Ordinal (or Interval if equal distances between points are assumed)
(iii) Interval/ratio
(iv) Interval/ratio
(v) Interval/ratio

Activity 19

1. Chi-squared test (data is nominal).
2. Wilcoxon or related t test.
3. Spearman or Pearson.
4. Mann-Whitney U test (data is ordinal)
5. Friedman or one-way anova for related samples.
6. Kruskal-Wallis or one-way anova for unrelated samples.

Activity 20

1. one-tailed (*more* effective).
2. two-tailed (*differentially* effective).
3. one-tailed (*fewer* complaints).
4. two-tailed (*difference* in strength)
5. one-tailed (*diminishes* vital capacity).

Converting the one-tailed hypotheses to two-tailed.
1. There is a difference in the effectiveness of praise as a motivator when used in a group or a 1–1 situation.
2. There is a difference in the number of complaints made by patients who attend either for rigorous exercise regimes or heat treatment in back schools.
3. The application of lumbar traction alters vital capacity.

Converting the two-tailed hypotheses to one-tailed.
1. Paraffin wax is more (less) effective than hot soaks as a preparation for mobilising exercises in post-fracture patients.
2. Strength of muscle contraction in a selected muscle group is reduced (increased) more by 2 minutes infrared radiation than by 2 minutes specific warm-up.

Activity 21

1. (i) $p < 0.025$ significant
   (ii) $p < 0.005$ significant
   (iii) $p = 0.02$ significant
   (iv) p is *greater than* 0.05, and is therefore not significant.
   (v) $p < 0.001$ significant
   (vi) $p < 0.05$ significant
2. $\chi^2 = 9.6; p < 0.01$

   Using the McNemar test ($\chi^2 = 9.6$) the results were significant ($p < 0.01$ (one-tailed). These results suggest that providing information about the reasons for changing on-call duty hours significantly alters physiotherapists' views in favour of the change.

Activity 22

1.

Subject	Condition A	Condition B	d	Rank
1	10	9	+1	3.5
2	8	9	−1	3.5
3	9	7	+2	7
4	6	7	−1	3.5
5	5	4	+1	3.5
6	8	3	+5	11
7	7	6	+1	3.5
8	9	9	0	omit
9	9	6	+3	8
10	5	6	−1	3.5
11	7	3	+4	9.5
12	8	4	+4	9.5

2. (i) $p < 0.05$ significant
    (ii) $p < 0.01$ significant
    (iii) $p < 0.025$ significant
    (iv) $p < 0.01$ significant
    (v) $p < 0.1$ not significant
    (vi) $p < 0.05$ significant
    (vii) $p = 0.01$ significant
    (viii) $p < 0.01$ significant
3. $T = 0$
   $N = 9$
   $p < 0.005$, one-tailed

Using a Wilcoxon on the data $(T = 0, N = 9)$ the results were found to be significant at $p < 0.005$ (one-tailed). These results support the hypothesis that traction is significantly more effective than surgical collars in the treatment of cervical spondylosis.

Activity 23

1. (i) $p = 0.033$ significant
    (ii) $p < 0.02$ significant
    (iii) $p < 0.072$ not significant
    (iv) $p < 0.001$ significant
    (v) $p < 0.008$ significant

(If you got any of these wrong, or are confused about the answers, do check that you were using the correct table, see p. 119).

2. $\chi r^2 = 2.658$, $p < 0.305$; not significant

Using a Friedman test to analyse the data, the results were not significant $(\chi r^2 = 2.658, p < 0.305)$. This suggests that there is no significant difference in the tone of the quadraceps muscle between Asian, Caucasian and West Indian children. The null hypothesis can therefore be accepted.

Activity 24

1. (i) $p < 0.01$ significant
    (ii) $p = 0.05$ significant
    (iii) $p < 0.05$ significant
    (iv) $p < 0.001$ significant
    (v) p is greater than 0.05 and is therefore not significant.

2. $L = 105$ $p < 0.05$

Using the Page's L trend test to analyse the data, the results were significant $(L = 105, p < 0.05)$. These results support the experimental hypothesis that hydrotherapy is more effective than exercise, which in turn is more effective than massage in the mobilisation of lower limbs paralysed following a stroke.

Activity 25

(i) $p < 0.025$ significant
(ii) $p < 0.1$ not significant
(iii) $p < 0.01$ significant
(iv) $p < 0.01$ significant
(v) $p < 0.02$ significant

2. $t = 2.362$; df $= 11$; $p < 0.025$

Using a related t test to analyse the data, the results were found to be significant at $p < 0.025$ ($t = 2.362$, df $= 11$). This suggests that student physiotherapists with 'A'-level physics do better in their 1st year theory exam marks, than students without 'A'-level physics. The null hypothesis can therefore be rejected in favour of the experimental hypothesis.

Activity 26

1. (i) $p < 0.05$ significant
    (ii) $p < 0.01$ significant
    (iii) p is greater than 0.05 and is therefore not significant
    (iv) $p < 0.025$ significant
    (v) $p < 0.05$ significant
    (iv) $p < 0.025$ significant

2.

Source of variation in scores	SS	df	MS	F ratios
Variation in scores *between conditions*	31.445	2	15.723	3.529
Variation in scores *between subjects*	76.278	5	15.256	3.424
Variation in scores due to random *error*	44.555	10	4.456	
Total	152.278	17		

F ratio $= 3.529$; df_{bet} $= 2$; df_{error} $= 10$; p is not significant.
F ratio$_{subj}$ $= 3.424$; df_{subj} $= 5$; df_{error} $= 10$
$p < 0.05$; significant

These results suggest that there is no significant effect from the different types of therapy used, but that the sets of matched subjects *were* significantly different from one another, and were therefore an atypical sample. These results can be expressed in the following way:

Using a one-way anova for related samples, no significant differences were found between the three treatment conditions ($F = 3.529$, $df_{bet} = 2$, $df_{error} = 10$). This suggests that the type of therapy used on hip replacement patients has no significant effect on mobility after 1 week. However, significant differences were found between the sets of matched subjects, ($F = 3.424$, $df_{subj} = 5$, $df_{error} = 10$, $p < 0.05$). This indicates that the subject sample was an atypical group and may represent a flaw in the sampling procedure. The null hypothesis must therefore be accepted.

Activity 27

1. Comparisons:
   a. *Condition 1* (seminar) × *Condition 2* (tutorial)
      $(F^1 = (C - 1)\ 3.34 = 10.02)$
      $F = 6.996\ p > 0.05$ not significant

   This suggests that the tutorial method is not significantly more effective than seminars in promoting understanding among a group of physiotherapy students.

   b. *Condition 1* (seminar) × *Condition 3* (lecture)
      $(F^1 = (C - 1)\ 3.34 = 10.02)$
      $F = 0.485$; not significant

   This suggests that there is no difference in the effectiveness of seminar or lecture methods in developing understanding among physiotherapy students.

   c. *Condition 1* (seminar) × *Condition 4* (reading)
      $(F^1 = (C - 1)\ 14.24 = 12.72)$
      $F = 15.194\ p < 0.025$ significant

   This suggests that seminars are more effective than reading for developing understanding in a group of physiotherapy students.

   d. *Condition 2* (tutorial) × *Condition 3* (lecture)
      $(F^1 = (C - 1)\ 3.34 = 10.02)$
      $F = 11.163,\ p < 0.05$, significant

   These results indicate that the tutorial is more effective than lectures in developing student physiotherapists' understanding.

   e. *Condition 2* (tutorial) × *Condition 4* (reading)
      $(F^1\ (C - 1)\ 9.73 = 29.19)$
      $F = 42.810\ p < 0.001$, significant

   These results suggest that tutorials are significantly more effective than reading for developing understanding in a group of physiotherapy students.

   f. *Condition 3* (lecture) × *Condition 4* (reading)
      $(F^1\ (C - 1)\ 3.34 = 10.02)$
      $F = 10.252\ p < 0.05$, significant

   These results suggest that lectures are significantly more effective than reading in promoting physiotherapy sutdents' understanding.

Activity 28

1. (i) $p < 0.025$ significant
    (ii) $p < 0.02$ significant
    (iii) $p = 0.05$ significant
    (iv) p is greater than 0.10 and is therefore not significant
    (v) $p < 0.005$ significant
2. χ^2 8.377 df $= 1, p < 0.005$
   Using a χ^2 to analyse the data ($\chi^2 = 8.377$, df $= 1$) the results were signifi-

cant ($p < 0.005$, one-tailed). This means that the null hypothesis can be rejected and that teachers of physiotherapy are more likely to study for Open University degree courses than clinically-based physiotherapists.

Activity 29

1. (i) $p < 0.05$ significant
    (ii) $p = 0.05$ significant
    (iii) $p < 0.01$ significant
    (iv) $p < 0.005$ significant
    (v) $p < 0.05$ significant
    (vi) p is larger than 0.10 and is therefore not significant.
2. $U = 45$, $p < 0.01$, one-tailed test

Using a Mann-Whitney U test on the data ($U = 45$, $N_1 = 14$, $N_2 = 14$) the results were found to be significant at $p < 0.01$ for a one-tailed hypothesis. This suggests that the experimental hypothesis has been supported and that paraffin wax is more effective than a hot soak as a preparation for mobilising exercises on post-fracture patients.

Activity 30

1. (i) $p < 0.046$ significant
    (ii) $p < 0.049$ significant
    (iii) $p < 0.05$ significant
    (iv) $p < 0.011$ significant
    (v) $p < 0.01$ significant
    (vi) p is larger than 0.05, and is therefore not significant.
2. $H = 6.26$, $N_1 = 5$, $N_2 = 5$, $N_3 = 5$ $p < 0.049$

Using a Kruskal-Wallis test on the data ($H = 6.26$, $N_1 = 5$, $N_2 = 5$, $N_3 = 5$), the results were found to be significant ($p < 0.049$ for a two-tailed test). This suggests that the three methods of giving postnatal exercise instructions are differentially effective. This means the null hypothesis can be rejected and the experimental hypothesis supported.

Activity 31

1. (i) $p < 0.01$ significant
    (ii) p is greater than 0.05 and so the results are not signficant
    (iii) $p < 0.05$ significant
    (iv) $p < 0.01$ significant
    (v) $p < 0.05$ significant
    (vi) p is greater than 0.05 and therefore the results are not significant.
2. $A = 128$, $B = 192$, $S = 64$, $C = 3$, $n = 8$, $p < 0.05$

Using a Jonckheere trend test to analyse the results ($S = 64$, $C = 3$, $n = 8$) the results were found to be significant ($p < 0.05$, one-tailed). This suggests that there is a significant trend in the probability of keeping outpatients' appointments, according to social class, with social class 3 being the most likely to keep them, followed by social class 2, and finally social class 4. The null hypothesis can be rejected.

Activity 32

1. (i) p is greater than 10% and so the results are not significant.
    (ii) $p < 0.05$ significant
    (iii) $p < 0.05$ significant
    (iv) p is greater than 5% and so the results are not significant.
    (v) $p < 0.02$ significant
2. $\chi^2 = 5.095$, df $= 2$, p is greater than 5% and so is not significant.
    Using an Extended χ^2 on the data, ($\chi^2 = 5.095$, df $= 2$) the results were found to be not significant (p is greater than 5%). Therefore the null hypothesis is accepted; there is no significant relationship between keeping an outpatients' appointment and ease of journey, using public transport.

Activity 33

1. (i) $p < 0.05$ significant
    (ii) $p < 0.02$ significant
    (iii) $p = 0.01$ significant
    (iv) p is larger than 5% and so the results are not significant.
    (v) $p < 0.01$ significant
2. $t = 2.43$; df $= 25$; $p < 0.025$
    Using an unrelated t test on the data ($t = 2.43$, df $= 25$), the results were significant ($p < 0.025$ for a one-tailed test). The null hypothesis can be rejected. This suggests that absenteeism is significantly greater among basic grade physiotherapists than among senior IIs.

Activity 34

1. (i) $p < 0.01$ significant
    (ii) $p < 0.001$ significant
    (iii) $p < 0.05$ significant
    (iv) $p < 0.01$ significant
2. $F = 2.171$, p is greater than 5% and is therefore not significant.

Source of:	SS	df	MS	F ratio
Variation due to treatment, i.e. *between* conditions	180.952	2	90.476	2.171
Variation due to random *error*	750	18	41.667	
Total	930.952	20		

Using a one-way anova for unrelated subject designs on the data ($F =$

2.171, $df_{bet} = 2$, $df_{error} = 18$) the results were found to be not significant (p is greater than 5%). This means that the null hypothesis must be accepted and that there is no relationship between the age of cystic fibrosis patients and the efficacy of clapping.

Activity 35

1. a. Comparison of 1975 and 1980
      $F = 4.982$
      p is not significant
      i.e. 'A'-level results were not significantly higher in 1980 than in 1975.
   b. Comparison of 1975 and 1985
      $F = 35.124$
      $p < 0.001$
      i.e. 'A'-level results were significantly higher in 1985 than in 1975.
   c. Comparison of 1980 and 1985
      $F = 13.649$
      $p < 0.01$
      i.e. 'A'-level results were significantly higher in 1985 than in 1980.

Activity 36

1. H_1 There is a relationship between the age of the patient and vital capacity.
   a. *Correlational Design*
      You would select one group of subjects who represented a whole range of ages (e.g. 15–65). You would then measure their vital capacities to see if there was any correlation between age and vital capacity.
   b. *Experimental Design*
      You have two possible options here.
      Firstly, you might select two groups of subjects one being at the young/ish end of the age range and the other being at the older end.

      Group 1   15–30 years (for example)
      Group 2   50–65 years (for example)

      You would measure their vital capacities to see if there was any *difference* between the groups.
      Alternatively, you might select a third group who represented a mid-age range thus:

      Group 1   15–25 years (for example)
      Group 2   35–45 years (for example)
      Group 3   55–65 years (for example)

      Again you would compare their vital capacities for differences between the groups.

Activity 37

1. $p < 0.01$
   $p =$ not significant
   $p = 0.02$
   $p =$ not significant
   $p < 0.005$
2. Results of the calculation of the Spearman rho:
   $r_s = -0.827$
   $p = < 0.01$ (two-tailed)
   Using a Spearman test on the data, $(r_s = -0.827, N = 10)$ the results were found to be significant ($p < 0.01$ for a two-tailed test). This suggests that there is a significant negative correlation between the length of lunch-break and professional competence. The null hypothesis can, therefore, be rejected.

Activity 38

1. (i) $p < 0.05$
   (ii) $p =$ not significant
   (iii) $p < 0.005$
   (iv) $p = 0.02$
   (v) $p < 0.001$
2. Results of the calculation of the Pearson product moment correlation:
   $r = +0.899$
   $p < 0.005$ (one-tailed)
   Using a Pearson product moment correlation test on the data ($r = +0.899$, df $= 6$), the results were found to be significant ($p < 0.005$, for a one-tailed test). This means that there is a significant positive correlation between students' marks on their 1st year exam and their averaged continuous assessment mark throught the year. The null hypothesis can therefore be rejected.

Activity 39

1. (i) $p < 0.05$
   (ii) p is greater than 5% and is therefore not significant.
   (iii) $p < 0.01$
   (iv) $p < 0.01$
   (v) p is greater than 5% and is therefore not significant.
2. Results of the calculation of the Kendall coefficient of concordance
   $s = 77, W = 0.616$
   $p < 0.05$
   Using the Kendall coefficient of concordance on the data ($s = 77, W = 6.61, n = 5, N = 4$) the results were found to be significant ($p < 0.05$ for a one-tailed test). This suggests that there is significant agreement on knee-movement when measured by a goniometer. The null hypothesis can be rejected.

Activity 40

1. $a = 0.939$, $b = 0.47$
    a. This patient would be in labour for 11.749 hours.
    b. This patient would be in labour for 8.459 hours.
    c. This patient would be in labour for 14.569 hours.

References

Chalmers A F 1983 What is this thing called science? Open University Press, Milton Keynes

Ferguson GA 1976 Statistical analysis in psychology and education. McGraw-Hill Kogakusha, Tokyo

Gardener G 1978 Social surveys for social planners. Open University Press, Milton Keynes

Greene J, D'Oliveira M 1982 Learning to use statistical tests in psychology. Open University Press, Milton Keynes

McNemar Q 1962 Psychological statistics. Wiley, New York

Siegel S 1956 Nonparametric statistics for the behavioural sciences. McGraw-Hill Kogakusha, Tokyo·

Index